Feasting on the Banquet of His Presence: Weight Loss God's Way

by Michele Sexton

Feasting on the Banquet of His Presence

Sometimes, in my quiet time with Him, the Lord gives me just "morsels" of Himself – enough to be an "appetizer" for me, teasing my appetite into wanting more of Him.

Other times He feeds me the "entrée;" straight up, no preliminaries, just the main "meat" with no fancy "hors-d'oeuvres" to distract me from His filling.

Sometimes just knowing He is there, the knowledge of His interest in my life, and the fact that He loves me is like the sweetest, richest "dessert" I could savor.

Ah, but sometimes His presence falls all around me, enveloping me in the loving arms of His embrace, as I dwell in His living Word and feast on the banquet of His presence.

It is at those times that I am fed the "living manna" and could never want for more.

--Michele Sexton

"How priceless is your unfailing love! Both high and low among men find refuge in the shadow of your wings. They feast on the abundance of your house; you give them drink from your river of delights." (Psa. 36:7-8)

4

Dedication

To all those people who have struggled with being overweight, unsuccessful dieting, and low self-esteem because of it – May God show you a better way.

Part One: Introduction

I have struggled with weight my entire life. For most of my life, I have been overweight. At only five feet tall, even the slightest bit of weight gain would show on my body.

It wasn't just the extra weight – it was the way my clothes fit. It was so frustrating, all those years, not being able to wear the clothes I wanted to wear; but, instead, having to wear clothes that hid my fat.

I tried every fad diet that came along – especially the ones that promised rapid weight loss. I wanted that boost in self-esteem that comes from being thinner.

However, I failed on every diet I ever tried.

It wasn't that I didn't lose weight, it was that I couldn't keep the weight off. And that was so frustrating – even depressing. When depressed, unfortunately, I would eat even more, thus continuing the cycle.

My life has been a pattern in yo-yo weight gain and loss. I even had two sets of clothes – my fat clothes and my thin clothes. Of course, I didn't get to wear my thin clothes very often.

I found that my self-image was directly related to my weight – in other words, if I was thinner, I felt better about myself; however, when I would inevitably gain the weight back, I felt terrible about myself again.

Finally, I gave in.

And I ballooned up to 165 pounds. Now, remember, we are talking about 165 pounds on a five-foot frame. I was then in size 14 clothes.

My self-esteem plummeted, and I lost hope that I would ever be "thin and beautiful."

Then, one miraculous day, God showed me how to eat *His* way, and I lost 60 pounds in nine months, going from a size 14 to a size 4.

How did I do it? Well, that's what this book is about.

And since Acts 10:34 says that *"God is no respecter of persons,"* what He did for me, He can do for you, too!

Part Two: The Truth

The truth is that God never meant us all to be perfect size 2 bodies in small frames and looking like the models on television and in magazines.

1 Peter 3:3-4 says, *"Your beauty should not come from outward adornment... Instead, it should be that of your inner self, the unfading beauty of a gentle and quiet spirit, which is of great worth in God's sight."*

The truth is that God is more concerned with your *inner self* - with your spirit - than he is with your outward appearance.

1 Samuel 16:7 says, *"...The Lord does not look at the things man looks at. Man looks at the outward appearance, but the Lord looks at the heart."*

The truth is that God is more concerned with the state of your heart than the size of your clothes.

On the other hand, He never meant for you to be overweight, either.

God calls overeating (or not eating right) *gluttony*, and He considers it a sin. Now, God has no sliding scale for sin – sin is sin in God's eyes, and we must repent for it.

Which is why the world's way of dieting is doomed to failure. You must acknowledge your sin and repent from it before you can be delivered from it.

However, once that has happened, and that sin is gone from your life, your weight loss can be permanent.

You have to have a change of heart before you can have a change of body.

Part Three: Eating Healthy vs. Dieting

With that heart change must also come a change in your thought patterns.

It's a matter of eating healthy vs. dieting. Eating healthy is a lifestyle change and a lifestyle choice – it is much more permanent than a diet.

That's why there are lasting results.

That's why fad diets come and go, but healthy eating can remain.

You just have to change the way you look at things related to food.

God meant food to be to the nourishment of our bodies. It is the world that perverted it into a lust for satisfaction.

For me, that lust for food (that sin of gluttony) carried over into the lust for the "perfect body," the "perfect shape," and later even for the "perfect clothes."

Models starve themselves to look the way that they do. God never meant for us to starve ourselves or to go on crash diets.

God meant food for our nourishment and enjoyment – and when you learn to eat

11

healthy instead of dieting, you will enjoy food again.

Eating God's way is not a matter of depriving yourself of any good thing. It is a matter of choosing those things which are good and that will satisfy your hunger, that's all.

Again, eating food is for the satisfaction of hunger, not lust or gluttony.

Part Four: Making Changes

Eating God's way is a matter of making good changes and good choices.

The first thing I did was to cut out all red meat. Red meat is full of fat, and even makes you *feel* heavy after you eat it.

Chicken and fish are much healthier for you.

Which isn't to say that I didn't eat the occasional steak, because I did. But the emphasis is on *occasional*.

Then I basically cut out starches, like bread, biscuits, and potatoes.

When I did eat bread, I chose a whole-grain or wheat bread, and I ate it in moderation.

That's the difference between the world's way of dieting and God's way of healthy eating – the world would have you cut out everything you enjoy eating, thinking that you'll never be able to eat it again.

Although there were some things I needed to cut out of my diet, other things I was able to still eat in moderation.

The main thing is not to eat in excess.

Believe me, I did not want to give up my French Vanilla creamer for my morning coffee. So I didn't – I just replaced it with the fat-free version.

I love butter. So, rather than go without the taste of it, I replaced it with a butter substitute, and I used that in a spray, which means I used less of it, while still enjoying the taste of butter on my food.

Lest you believe that my food was bland, I'll give you a big hint right now: McCormick Season-All. It is the only seasoning I use on my food, and I use it on everything! It is especially flavorful on fish and chicken.

I began to make other changes as well.

I ate more fresh fruits and vegetables, and added nuts (in moderation) to my diet, especially natural almonds, which are very good for you.

Steamed fresh vegetables replaced frozen or canned vegetables in my diet. With a few sprays of my butter replacement, they were delicious!

I added dried fruits and nuts to my salads and used a flavored salad dressing (Fat-Free Raspberry Vinaigrette is my favorite), again, in a spray version so I would use less of it.

Just like some people like "everything pizza," I like "everything salad." If you put enough fruits, nuts, and fresh cut vegetables in it, an "everything salad" is a meal unto itself!

I stopped eating fried foods, and baked the food instead.

I definitely cut out fast food right away – you would not believe how fattening some of that food is! Although it may temporarily satisfy your hunger, it is not a healthy way in which to do it.

Again, it is a "quick fix" rather than a healthy choice.

I exchanged fattening foods for low-fat or fat-free wherever I could as well.

I replaced canned soups (high in sodium) and, instead, made wonderfully tasting soups out of any fresh vegetable I had on hand, combined with chicken broth and any leftover chicken I might have. Soup can be very filling and not very fattening.

I replaced some meals with yogurt smoothies (liquid yogurt).

I did not (and still do not) drink any soda. I drink only water, and of that I drink six 8-oz. glasses a day.

Water not only satisfies your thirst, but also cleanses away toxins and fat from your body.

So you can see that my eating just became a matter of healthy choices and replacements.

The last thing I did was to stay under 1000 calories per day. Now, that's for my size and weight, so yours may be 1200 or 1500 calories, depending on what your doctor says.

Part Five: The Rules

Since we are so used to "dieting" the world's way, we are bound to expect "rules" that govern that diet.

Ok, here are the rules:

1. Eat only when you're hungry (your stomach should tell you, not your head).

2. Eat only what you are hungry for (or else you will never be satisfied).

3. Eat everything in moderation or less (even the occasional dessert).

4. Stop eating when you are full (don't worry if there is still food on your plate).

5. Supplement your diet with a good multi-vitamin, B-complex (good for stress), and Omega-3 Fatty Oils (good for your heart).

6. Drink six 8-oz. glasses of water each day.

7. Exercise for 30 minutes, three times a week, even if it is just walking.

That's it! Just SEVEN rules! Do you think you can handle that?

I guess I would add an eighth rule to that, though: Don't feel guilty!

If you splurge once in a while, don't feel guilty about it. Just go back to eating your regular healthy diet the next day.

When I used to diet, the first thing I wanted was a candy bar, thinking I would never be able to eat one again.

I still love chocolate. Only now, I can eat just a half a candy bar and save the rest for another time.

Usually, though, I satisfy my craving for something sweet by eating a wholesome granola bar or some dried fruit.

I still love pizza. Only now, instead of three pieces, I only eat one.

Remember, everything in moderation.

Part Six: Feeding Your Spirit as Well as Your Body

Making good choices for your body is not enough. You also need to feed your spirit.

You need to be balanced: physically, mentally, emotionally, and spiritually.

Physically – exercise just 30 minutes, three times a week, even if it's just walking.

Mentally – make sure you do things that challenge your mind, like: work, reading, and learning new things.

Emotionally – try to keep your stress levels to a minimum, and make sure you have a good support system of people who care about you. Remember to relax and to do things you enjoy as well.

Spiritually – feed your spirit as much as you feed your body to stay spiritually fit.

Staying spiritually fit is the most important thing. Without it, the rest won't work.

That's why what follows is a 12-week daily devotional to inspire and encourage you on your journey to a healthier body and a better way to eat.

This devotional will help you to stay grounded in the Word, and to remember that God is with you on this journey.

12-Week
Devotional Journal
for

Feasting on the
Banquet
of His Presence

WEEK ONE
DAY ONE

"Then Jacob made a vow, saying, 'If God will be with me and will watch over me on this journey I am taking and will give me food to eat and clothes to wear so that I return safely to my father's house, then the Lord will be my God and this stone that I have set up as a pillar will be God's house, and of all that you give me I will give you a tenth."

--Gen. 28:20-22

Life is a journey through the desert of your past and present – not just eating habits, but also other things that need to die in the desert in you, just like Jacob.

Before he even left, he was trusting God for his food and clothing. He didn't take any food *with* him! He trusted God to give it to him when it was time.

Before I was convicted of my eating problem, I would not even venture out of my house without at least a candy bar in my purse, for fear that I would be some place where (God forbid) I would not have access to food when I needed it.

Food was such a stronghold of comfort for me, like my small son taking his "blankie" on a journey.

God would not take you on a journey for which He has not already gone before you and paved the way and, if He goes before you, He has already provided for your needs.

"Do not be like them, for your Father knows what you need before you ask him," says Matthew 6:8.

Let us, like Jacob, trust our Lord to meet all our needs, until we, too, *"return safely to [our] father's house."*

Dear Lord, help me to trust You to provide for all my needs, no matter how long the journey that stretches before me. Amen.

WEEK ONE
DAY TWO

"The priest is to sprinkle the blood against the altar of the Lord at the entrance to the Tent of Meeting and burn the fat as an aroma pleasing to the Lord."

--Lev. 17:6

Don't we all wish we could take this verse literally, and burn our fat, too! But why couldn't it be taken that way?

If we believe 2Corinthians 2:15, which says, *"For we are to God the aroma of Christ among those who are being saved and those who are perishing..."* then why wouldn't "burning the fat" *be* a pleasing aroma to the Lord?

For the burning off of the fat on your body would be out of obedience to the Lord – and obedience is *definitely* an *"aroma pleasing to the Lord."*

The only way we can be truly obedient in this, however, is to quit indulging in the sins of the flesh (eating as the world eats).

Leviticus 17:7 says, *"They must no longer offer any of their sacrifices to the goat idols to whom they prostitute themselves.*

This is to be a lasting ordinance for them and for the generations to come."

Accepting being overweight, justifying your size or eating habits, blaming your parents for your size, making excuses for head hunger, ignoring the fact that you're still snacking – these are all sacrifices to the god of food and fleshly satisfactions!

Let us, instead, offer up to God the sacrifices of obedience, even in the "burning of our fat."

Dear Lord, I repent of these wrong sacrifices, and give my whole body as a sacrifice to You. Use me, Lord, to Your service, to Your glory, in a way that is pleasing to You. Amen.

WEEK ONE
DAY THREE

"You must not do as they do in Egypt, where you used to live, and you must not do as they do in the land of Canaan, where I am bringing you. Do not follow their practices. You must obey my laws and be careful to follow my decrees. I am the Lord your God. Keep my decrees and laws, for the man who obeys them will live by them. I am the Lord."

--Lev. 18:3-5

God gave the Israelites many laws in the desert – some that apply today, some that don't. However, I believe that this Scripture applies not only for today, but for us personally.

"You must not do as they did in Egypt..." (the world, with all its man-made rules and diets), *"...where you used to live..."* (you have come *out* of the world – you don't walk in its ways any more).

"Do not follow their practices." (You are no longer to eat as the world eats or dictates that you eat).

"I am the Lord your God." (Seek God *first* – make *Him* your priority.)

"You must obey my laws..." (*obedience* is the key to victory) *"...and be careful to follow my decrees"* (don't let your guard down – don't give in to disobedience).

"Keep my decrees and laws..." (do it God's way and not your own way), *"...for the man who obeys them..."* (who continues to walk in obedience) *"...will live by them."* (it will eventually become second nature – you *will* walk in victory over food).

"I am the Lord." (Jesus is your Lord, *not* food).

Dear Lord, help me not to follow the ways of the world, but only to follow after you, to seek Your face and to walk in Your ways. Help me to keep these laws which You have set before me. Amen.

WEEK ONE
DAY FOUR

"Therefore go and make disciples of all nations, baptizing them in the name of the Father and of the Son and of the Holy Spirit, and teaching them to obey everything I have commanded you. And surely I am with you always, to the very end of the age."

--Matt. 28:19-20

God considered obedience so important, He even included it in the Great Commission!

However, this verse also shows that obedience is not something that comes naturally or easily; rather, that it must be learned, and that someone commissioned by Christ must teach them.

God first puts someone through the desert of testing (whether food or another area) so that when they have overcome that area through obedience, they can then go teach others how to overcome it also.

Jesus told it to Peter (Simon) this way in Luke 22:31-32, *"Simon, Simon, Satan has asked to sift you as wheat. But I have prayed for you, Simon, that your faith may not fail. And when you have turned back, strengthen your brothers."*

Consider then, that your own desert of testing is not just important for you, but for all the others you will then strengthen after you have succeeded.

Dear Lord, help me to remember that my obedience is not only important for myself, but for those others who will follow after me. Give me the courage and the strength I need to endure this time of being sifted. Amen.

WEEK ONE
DAY FIVE

"They must be holy to their God and must not profane the name of their God. Because they present the offerings made to the Lord by fire, the food of their God, they are to be holy."

--Lev. 21:6

"Regard them as holy, because they offer up the food of your God. Consider them holy, because I the Lord am holy – I who make you holy."

--Lev. 21:8

What is "the food of God?"

Jesus' food was to do the will of the Father. He also says that only those who do the will of the Father will enter into the kingdom of heaven (Matthew 7:21).

But what about God?

God's food was the burnt offerings. He is fed when we put to death (burn forever) our sinful nature – when we die to self so that He may live (in us).

Today we live by grace, not under the law; and, obviously, we no longer make burnt offering for our sin.

What, then, are the sacrifices pleasing to God today?

"You do not delight in sacrifice, or I would bring it; you do not take pleasure in burnt offerings. The sacrifices of God are a broken spirit; a broken and contrite heart, O God, you will not despise." (Psalms 51:16-17)

It is only by coming to God truly repentant, in brokenness of spirit, that He can begin to bind up our broken lives and truly have His way.

Dear Lord, help me to submit to You out of a broken and contrite heart. As I sacrifice food, and the bondage to it, to You, I ask You to make me holy in obedience to You. Amen.

WEEK ONE
DAY SIX

"Then the word of the Lord came to Jonah a second time: 'Go to the great city of Nineveh and proclaim to it the message I give you.' Jonah obeyed the word of the Lord and went to Nineveh. Now Nineveh was a very important city – a visit required three days."

--Jon. 3:1-3

How many of you are going through your N-teenth time of trying to lose weight?

It is encouraging to know that we are not the first ones to have to go through something more than once to get it right! The first time God spoke to Jonah, Jonah decided to do it his own way. Well, we all know about how he ended up inside the whale's belly!

Many of us also have to end up "inside a big fish" (our own bodies?) before we realize that our way doesn't work.

It is only after a second (or third) try that we submit our wills out of obedience to God and, like Jonah, go where the Lord will send us. Even if it *is* into the desert of testing.

Praise the Lord, that He is "the God of second chances!"

When we submit to Him, He will do for us what He did for the people of Nineveh:

"When God saw what they did and how they turned from their evil ways, he had compassion and did not bring upon them the destruction he had threatened." (Jonah 3:10)

Dear Lord, I praise You that You are the God of second chances. Help me to submit my will to You so that I will not need yet another chance. Amen.

WEEK ONE
DAY SEVEN

"If you remain hostile toward me and refuse to listen to me, I will multiply your afflictions seven times over, as your sins deserve."

--Lev. 26:21

"When I cut off your supply of bread, ten women will be able to bake your bread in one oven, and they will dole out the bread by weight. You will eat, but you will not be satisfied."

--Lev. 26:26

God talks about punishment for disobedience in Leviticus 26:14-46.

It is surprising that one of the punishments relates to food, in that when we are disobedient in the way of food, we will eat but will not be satisfied.

Surprising, yes. But very true, as many of us who have struggled with being overweight have found out many times over. Those times we eat out of only perceived (head) hunger (and not *real* stomach hunger), we really are not satisfied.

On the other hand, when the people listened to Jesus and were obedient to God, Jesus Himself broke the bread and fed them, and *"they all ate and were satisfied..."* (Mark 6:42)

We need to learn to put away our hostility toward God, and be obedient to doing things His way instead of our own.

It is only by listening to His "still small voice" that we learn to hear, trust, and obey in the way of food, as in all areas of our lives.

Dear Lord, I repent of my hostility toward You. I know that my way doesn't work. I pray that You would help me to do things Your way, to be satisfied with Your food. Amen.

WEEK TWO
DAY ONE

"Then, because so many people were coming and going that they did not even have a chance to eat, he said to them, 'Come with me by yourselves to a quiet place and get some rest.' So they went away by themselves in a boat to a solitary place."

--Mk. 6:31-32

"After leaving them, he went up on a mountainside to pray."

--Mk. 6:46

At times our lives are too busy, to the point of being overwhelming. At these times it is not only desirable, but necessary, to set aside quiet time to be with the Lord, to pray, and to get some rest. Even Jesus did this.

Too many of us have been caught in the trap of eating in a rush, whatever was available, whenever it was available, just because we were "too busy;" or of skipping meals, only to "double-up" on the next meal.

This trick of the enemy has been very effective in the past. But no longer!

Jesus Himself commands us to come with him to a place where things are quieter, slower; where there is all the time we need to regroup, to be refreshed, and to be in fellowship with Him.

The world has become a clamor of sin and degradation – the enemy speaks loudly in the media, in the world outside our homes, in the workplace... yet the Lord speaks softly in the midst of it all.

We need to take time away from the rush of the world to be quiet, in order to hear our own bodies speaking to us as far as *real* hunger, but also to hear the "still small voice" of our of Lord as He speaks to us about other areas of our lives in which we need to be obedient.

Dear Lord, help me to make it a priority to set aside quiet time to be with You. I need to hear Your voice speaking softly in the midst of the world's clamor. Amen.

WEEK TWO
DAY TWO

"Jesus looked at him and loved him. 'One thing you lack,' he said. 'Go, sell everything you have and give to the poor, and you will have treasure in heaven. Then come, follow me.' At this the man's face fell. He went away sad, because he had great wealth."

--Mk. 10:21-22

Why does it say, *"Jesus looked at him and loved him?"* Because Jesus was about to tell the rich man the hardest words of all.

He told him to give up that which he loved the most. For the rich man, that was his wealth. And he could not give it up for Christ, even for the promise of treasure in heaven, so he went away sad.

Jesus asks us all to give up that which we hold onto the tightest, anything we love more than Him.

If we cling too tightly to life itself, He says, *"The man who loves his life will lose it..."* even as He goes on to say, *"while the man who hates his life in this world will keep it for eternal life."* (John 12:25)

For those of us in a struggle with bondage to food, this is the very thing to which we hold the tightest... and this is the very thing that Jesus asks us to turn away from.

Even though He promises us treasure in Heaven (all the candy we want?), will we still hold onto our treasure of this life and walk away sad, as the rich man did, or will we choose the heavenly treasure of the obedient life?

Dear Lord, let me not walk away sad as the rich man did. Help me to be content with heavenly treasure, instead of worldly riches. Amen.

WEEK TWO
DAY THREE

"When the devil had finished all this tempting, he left him until an opportune time."

--Lk. 4:13

Luke 4:1-13 tells us about the temptation of Jesus.

How many of you, when you've heard that Jesus was tempted in *every* way just like us, scoffed and thought, "Yeah, but he sure didn't have to struggle with a weight problem!"

Ah, but think about this – the very first area of testing in Jesus' own desert *was* in the area of food!

Luke 4:1-2 tells us that, *"Jesus, full of the Holy Spirit, returned from the Jordan and was led by the Spirit in the desert, where for forty days he was tempted by the devil. He ate nothing during those days, and at the end of them he was hungry."*

The devil reminded Jesus that He (Jesus) could do anything He wanted – even to make the stones to become bread.

So we, also, have the freedom and the choice to eat whatever we want, whenever we want.

However, note Jesus' own response to this freedom: In verse 4, Jesus answered, *"It is written:*

'Man does not live on bread alone.'" We see here that even Jesus was obedient to God the Father!

If we are to be like Jesus, we must realize that He truly *was* tempted in every way as we are, even in the area of food. Even so, He remained obedient in spite of temptation.

Be aware, though, of this passage's last line (v.13): Satan only left Jesus for a more opportune time.

Do not believe for one minute that the enemy will leave you alone in this area – he won't! But if you remain obedient to God, you *will* be victorious over your enemy!

Dear Lord, help me to be more like Jesus, to be obedient to You, even as He was, and in this way be able to be victorious over my enemy. Amen.

WEEK TWO
DAY FOUR

"When I said, 'My foot is slipping,' your love, O Lord, supported me. When anxiety was great within me, your consolation brought joy to my soul."

--Psa. 94:18-19

How often do we try to do things our own way, only to find our feet slipping out from under us?

Usually it's because our self-will, or our pride, has once again reared its ugly head.

For the Bible says in the Old Testament that, *"Pride goes before destruction, a haughty spirit before a fall,"* (Proverbs 16:18) and is confirmed in the New Testament in 1Corinthians 10:12, which says: *"So, if you think you are standing firm, be careful that you don't fall."*

It is a mistake at any time to believe that we can conquer this desert on our own. As you begin to find success in weight loss God's way, it's easy to lose sight of the fact that it is only through *God's* working that you are finding success at all.

As Ephesians 2:8-9 tells us, *"For it is by grace you have been saved, through faith – and this not from yourselves, it is the gift of God – not by works, so that no one can boast."*

If you do see your feet begin to slip, remind yourself of where you were before trying to lose

43

weight God's way; the many man-made (self-made) ways that you tried to lose the weight.

Then also remind yourself how every one of them failed.

It is the grace of God that is teaching you how to lose weight God's way, and the love of God that will keep your foot from slipping.

Dear Lord, help me to stand on Your solid ground – keep my foot from slipping back into my own way. Amen.

WEEK TWO
DAY FIVE

"'Can anyone hide himself in secret places, so I shall not see him?' says the Lord; 'Do I not fill heaven and earth?' says the Lord."

--Jer. 23:24

What the NIV version of the Bible refers to as "disobedience" in places (Hebrews, for example), the KJV version refers to as "unbelief." How do these two terms coincide?

Our disobedience to God, not just in the area of food, but in any area, stems from our *unbelief* that He will do what He promised!

The affirmation is this, according to Psalms 145:13b, *"The Lord is faithful to all his promises and loving toward all he has made."* God has promised to bring us through this desert of testing with food, and He will! However, we have a responsibility as well: *"Be on your guard; stand firm in the faith; be men of courage; be strong. Do everything in love."* (1Corinthians 16:13-14)

If we do everything out of love for our Savior, we will be walking in obedience without the *effort* of walking in obedience. Love itself will direct our steps. And since love *"believes all things,"* (1Corinthians 13:7), it leaves no room for disobedience.

God has outlined His plan for our deliverance from bondage to food in His Word. We are no longer to eat "secret" foods in "secret" places (guiltily hidden from sight), or foods pre-determined by a man-made exchange list.

"Instead you are to eat them in the presence of the Lord your God at the place the Lord your God will choose..." says Deuteronomy 12:18.

If you are ashamed for God to see what you are eating, if you are afraid to eat it in His presence, then it is disobedience. Disobedience is sin, and you cannot hide your sin from God. And if it is not the place the Lord has chosen (i.e., the "when" of your eating), then it is disobedience – your head has decided to eat now, and not your stomach. This is eating *your* way, at *your* time/place, and *not* God's!

Coming into line with weight loss God's way means coming into line with God's design for our eating habits, as well as His overall design for our lives. We need to take God at His word – believe His promises to us – and not sacrifice obedience in our unbelief.

Dear Lord, forgive my unbelief. I repent of my disobedience to You, the sin of eating "secret" foods in "secret" places. Help me to learn Your ultimate plan for my eating, as well as for my life.

WEEK TWO
DAY SIX

"'What do you want me to do for you?' Jesus asked him. The blind man said, 'Rabbi, I want to see.' 'Go,' said Jesus, 'your faith has healed you.' Immediately he received his sight and followed Jesus along the road."

--Mk. 10:51-52

Mark 10:46-52 tells us the story of Blind Bartimaeus receiving his sight. His blindness was a handicap for him, one with which he had lived for a long time. A long time, until he heard of Jesus and then had the hope that he might not remain blind forever.

For many of us, our fat is like Bartimaeus' blindness. We have lived with it for a long time, without even the hope of not being fat forever. Yet now we do have hope – the same hope that Bartimaeus had! The hope that Jesus, in His compassion, will not pass us by and leave us in our handicap, but will do for us what He did for Bartimaeus.

We might even rewrite this passage as if Jesus were speaking to us: *"What do you want me to do for you'" Jesus asked you. You said, "Rabbi, I want to be thin." "Go," said Jesus, "your faith has healed you." Immediately you were thin and followed Jesus along the road.*

This might seem a bit unorthodox, but many people struggling with bondage to food feel that their weight is as much a handicap to them as blindness was to Bartimaeus.

Hoping against hope for deliverance from being overweight, we cling to the faith of Bartimaeus – the faith of one hoping against the odds that Jesus would have compassion and deliver them. We think, "If Bartimaeus' faith could heal him, then mine can heal me!"

Jesus said that if we had faith as small as a mustard seed, we could say to a mountain to be moved, and it would! With only that small amount of faith, let us trust Jesus to move this mountain. We say to this mountain of fat, "Be moved!"

Dear Lord, I need You to move this mountain for me – I can't do it myself. I feel so handicapped with all this extra weight – just as Bartimaeus did with his blindness. As he did, so do I trust You to heal and deliver me. Amen.

WEEK TWO
DAY SEVEN

"And he will go on before the Lord, in the spirit and power of Elijah, to turn the hearts of the fathers to their children and the disobedient to the wisdom of the righteous – to make ready a people prepared for the Lord."

--Lk. 1:17

Many of you have questioned why you've had to go through this struggle; why you were selected for the desert of testing, and why in this manner? Have you considered that you are not going through this struggle for yourself alone?

John the Baptist was sent before Jesus to turn *"the disobedient to the wisdom of the righteous."*

Paul said in 2Corinthians 5:21b that in Christ, *"...we might become the righteousness of God."* So if we, first, become righteous, through becoming obedient to Christ, we can then also turn the disobedient to the wisdom of the righteous.

How do we attain this *"wisdom of the righteous?"* How do any of us learn wisdom?

The Bible says in James 1:5, *"If any of you lack wisdom, he should ask God, who gives generously to all without finding fault, and it will be given to him."*

Through obedience, we are gaining righteousness. Through asking God, we will gain wisdom.

Why are you reading this book? You are reading it because you were looking for a better way to control your weight. You asked God for wisdom, and He is teaching you obedience.

You have desired to be closer to God, and He is taking you through this desert so that you might be made righteous. And what is His purpose for you in all this? *"To make ready a people prepared for the Lord."*

Dear Lord, I ask You for wisdom in this desert. I know I can't do this on my own. I know that righteousness can only come from You, and I need Your righteousness to point the way for others. Amen.

WEEK THREE
DAY ONE

"Whatever you have commanded us we will do, and wherever you send us we will go."

--Josh. 1:16

"Don't urge me to leave you or to turn back from you. Where you go I will go, and where you stay I will stay."

--Ruth 1:16

Both these verses are similar in their expression of obedience. In Joshua 1:16, we find the Israelites telling Joshua that they will do whatever he tells them to do. Their obedience stems from a willingness to follow him, as they had followed Moses before him.

In Ruth's case, however, as she is speaking to Naomi in Ruth 1:16, her obedience stems more from love than anything else.

What about you? Are you being obedient to God? And does that obedience stem from a willing heart, a servant's heart, so that out of *love* for Jesus you will follow Him wherever He leads you?

Or are you more like the Israelites, who only wanted to follow Joshua because they had followed Moses before him?

Are you looking for someone to lead you, or are you following Jesus, the Leader? Are you following in blind obedience, or the obedience that stems from love, like Ruth?

51

Jesus said in John 14:23a, *"If anyone loves me, he will obey my teaching."*

He also said in John 15:10, *"If you obey my commands, you will remain in my love, just as I have obeyed my Father's commands and remain in his love."*

Obedience and love go hand in hand. We must choose to follow Jesus out of love.

Dear Lord, help me to be obedient to Your commands; to follow You out of a heart of obedient love. Amen.

WEEK THREE
DAY TWO

"Blessed is she who has believed that what the Lord has said to her will be accomplished!"

--Lk. 1:45

Has God spoken to your heart...given you a promise?

Has He shown you visions of what you will look like when you are thin?

Has He told you what He wants to do through you? And have you listened? Do you believe Him? Or do you just *want* to believe Him, but secretly (fearfully) doubt in your heart that you ever really will be thin?

Like the father in Mark 9:24, do you also say, *"Lord, I believe; forgive my unbelief!"*

Many of us face obstacles that we can see no earthly way of overcoming. It is difficult sometimes to believe in God's intercession in the small things that concern us.

But we must believe that *"God is faithful to all his promises and loving toward all he has made"* (Psalms 145:13), and that He *is* concerned about us, and *will* intercede in our affairs, if we will but believe.

Jesus said in Mark 9:23, *"Everything is possible for him who believes."*

Even if you only have a small amount of faith, you can stand on God's Word, claiming the promise of Luke 1:37, that *"...nothing is impossible with God."*

Then you, too, will be blessed for believing that what the Lord said to you will be accomplished!

Dear Lord, I do believe that nothing is impossible with You. I trust in Your promise to me, and believe that what You said, You will do. Amen.

WEEK THREE
DAY THREE

"He holds victory in store for the upright, he is a shield to those whose walk is blameless, for he guards the course of the just and protects the way of his faithful ones."

--Prov. 2:7-8

Have you become discouraged in the desert?

Do you find yourself looking at how long the road stretches before you – how far you have yet to travel?

Could it be that, even in some small way, you have gone back to your own way?

Could it be that, even for a short time, you have taken your eyes off Jesus?

Discouragement creeps in when we focus on how far we have yet to go, instead of how far we have already come. It will also creep in when, even inadvertently, we once again try to do things our own way.

Only in true and absolute obedience to God will our walk be found blameless, for the Lord Himself will order our steps. Then *He* will be our shield... *He* will guard our course... and *He* will protect our way.

When we give ourselves over to the Lord wholeheartedly, submit to Him out of obedience, and commit our ways to Him, He *will* give us victory!

Proverbs 16:3 says, *"Commit to the Lord whatever you do, and your plans will succeed."*

Only by doing this will you achieve any lasting success, not only in your weight loss, but in your Christian walk as well.

Dear Lord, I commit my way to You – I give you this journey, and pray that You would order my steps throughout it. Amen.

WEEK THREE
DAY FOUR

"When she heard in Moab that the Lord had come to the aid of his people by providing food for them, Naomi and her daughters-in-law prepared to return home from there."

--Ruth 1:6

In this passage in the Book of Ruth, we learn that there had been a famine in the land of Judah.

Because of the famine, Naomi's husband led her to the land of Moab, thinking that things would be better for them there. After his death, Naomi heard about what the Lord was doing back in Judah, and *"prepared to return home from there."*

How many of us, also, when confronted with a "famine" (temporary loss of *any* provision from God) in our lives, look to see that "the grass is always greener on the other side of the fence," like Naomi did?

So many of us, facing difficult trials and temptations, choose to run from them; only to find out that God's provision really had been in the midst of the trial itself.

In this passage from Ruth, *back home* is where *"...the Lord had come to the aid of his people by providing food for them."*

How many of us, when facing *our* "famine," try to provide for ourselves (do it our own way), only to find out that God had already made a way (*His* way) to provide for us?

When faced with a "famine" (temporary loss of *any* provision from God), you must learn to resist the temptation to flee the situation – to run away – to seek greener pastures.

If you will remain in the situation, you will find that "...*my God will meet all your needs according to his glorious riches in Christ Jesus.*" (Philippians 4:19)

Dear Lord, I praise You, my Jehovah-Jireh, my Provider, who provides for all my needs. Help me to resist the temptation to flee the "famines" in my life, but instead to trust You for my provision. Amen.

WEEK THREE
DAY FIVE

"The Lord continued to appear at Shiloh, and there he revealed himself to Samuel through his word."

--1Sam. 3:21

Some of you still struggle with a daily devotional time, a time set aside to be alone with God and study His Word.

For some, it's a matter of "not enough hours in the day." To those people, I would say that if you would tithe the first 10% of your day, just like you do your money, God will increase the *time* you have, just like He does your finances!

Others struggle with the motivation to wake up each day and get into the Word. Those people I would encourage with the verse from 1Samuel 3:21.

If your desert walk is feeling pretty "dry" these days, let the Lord refresh you with His Word. He longs to reveal Himself to you today as much as He did to Samuel back then.

And how did He reveal himself? Through His Word!

A saying has been written that the Bible is God's love letter to us. If we are His bride, and He is our bridegroom (John 3:29), could it not be so?

As Isaiah 62:5 says, *"...as a bridegroom rejoices over his bride, so will your God rejoice over you."* And, if so, wouldn't you want to wake up each day excited about what your beloved has written to you that day?

If you will commit to tithing the first 10% of your day, even starting with only ten minutes each morning, you will find yourself "washed with the Word," and before long, ten minutes will not be enough!

Just like your morning shower cleans the outside of your body, so God's Word will clean and refresh the inside of your heart.

Dear Lord, I long to read Your Word as if it were Your love letter to me. Help me to set aside time each morning to spend with You. Amen.

WEEK THREE
DAY SIX

*"'But what about you?' he asked. 'Who do you say I
am?' Peter answered, 'The Christ of God."*

--Lk. 9:20

What about YOU? Who do *you* say He is?

Some in the crowd that day thought Jesus was
John the Baptist; others thought maybe Elijah; others
(and many people still today) believed He was just a
prophet. But as Jesus challenged Peter, so I challenge
you.

What about YOU? Who do *you* say He is?

If He is John, or Elijah, or a prophet, then He
has no power in your life today to deliver you from
bondage. *But...* if you can answer as Peter did, that He
is *"the Christ of God,"* then He is your deliverer.

"The Spirit of the Lord is upon me," Jesus said
in Luke 4:18-19, *"because he has anointed me to
preach good news to the poor. He has sent me to
proclaim freedom for the prisoners and recovery of
sight for the blind, to release the oppressed, to
proclaim the year of the Lord's favor."*

If you believe Jesus is *"the Christ of God,"* then
this is the Christ you serve! One who is big enough to
deliver you not only from bondage to food, but any
other stronghold that oppresses you or holds you
prisoner.

"What about you?" Jesus asks, *"Who do you say I am?"*

Whatever else He is to you, He must first be a very *personal* Christ.

Your relationship with Him must be an intimate one, as the Bride to the Bridegroom. Jesus does not ask what other people think of Him – only what YOU think of Him! And your answer must be, as Peter's, *"You are the Christ of God."*

Dear Lord, I do believe that You are the Christ of God. Set me free from bondage and release me from oppression, that I may serve You always, in freedom and in love. Amen.

WEEK THREE
DAY SEVEN

"Then he said to them all: 'If anyone would come after me, he must deny himself and take up his cross daily and follow me."

--Lk. 9:23

Most of us still struggle on a daily basis with one form of bondage or another – after all, none of us is perfect.

Even those of you who are having much success with weight loss God's way may still struggle with bondage in other areas.

Even as God delivers us from one area of bondage in our lives, it (too soon) seems that He just as quickly reveals another area of our lives that needs to be "cleaned up."

Sometimes we might even want to cry out, "Don't I get a break, Lord?"

God never said it would be easy. He did say it would be *daily*, though!

Every day, each of us must deny himself, take up his cross, and follow Jesus.

Each day that we purpose in our hearts to follow Jesus means that we try to be more like Him.

And His cross was certainly not easy to bear, nor did He cry out, "Don't I get a break, Lord?"

Jesus said in John 16:33, *"I have told you these things so that in me you may have peace. In this world you will have trouble. But take heart! I have overcome the world."*

Take heart, dear friend, for you do not bear your cross alone.

Dear Lord, help me to take up my cross daily and follow You. Help me to deny myself willingly, and to submit to Your deliverance. Amen.

WEEK FOUR
DAY ONE

"And the Lord told him: 'Listen to all that the people are saying to you; it is not you they have rejected, but they have rejected me as their king."

--1Sam. 8:7

When I first learned how to lose weight God's way, one of the areas in which I realized very quickly that I needed deliverance was fear of what other people thought of me; fear of rejection.

As I had gone up in size, so I had also gone down in witnessing. I had decided to be a "silent witness." Concerned that being overweight destroyed my witness about a Savior who could deliver from anything, I chose to be silent.

In repentance, I question myself, "How many lost opportunities? How many others could have been saved if I'd been less concerned about me and more concerned about their salvation? How many seeds did I not plant? How many people have perished because I was afraid to tell them of my King, for fear they'd reject *me*?

Samuel knew the discouragement of people's rejection, but when he prayed about it, God told him it wasn't Samuel that the people were rejecting, but God as their King.

Jesus knew rejection, too. He said in John 15:18, *"If the world hates you, keep in mind that it hated me first."*

Regardless of our "outward packaging," we MUST continue to tell others about the saving grace of Jesus – whether they accept us or reject us! Even as Jesus said, it is not us they are rejecting, but Him.

Jesus said in Luke 10:16 that *"he who listens to you listens to me; he who rejects you rejects me; but he who rejects me rejects him who sent me."*

Regardless of our size, regardless of our fear of rejection, regardless of concern about what other people think, we must never be afraid to speak the Word of God boldly.

Dear Lord, deliver me from my fears. Give me courage and boldness to tell others about You, regardless of whether they accept me or not. Amen.

WEEK FOUR
DAY TWO

"She had a sister called Mary, who sat at the Lord's feet listening to what he said. But Martha was distracted by all the preparations that had to be made. She came to him and asked, 'Lord, don't you care that my sister has left me to do the work by myself? Tell her to help me!' 'Martha, Martha,' the Lord answered, 'you are worried and upset about many things, but only one thing is needed. Mary has chosen what is better, and it will not be taken away from her."

--Lk. 10:39-42

Are you a Mary, who sits quietly at Jesus' feet, absorbing His teachings?

Or are you a Martha, distracted, *"worried and upset about many things?"*

Martha was so busy "doing works" for the Lord, while the only "work" Jesus wanted at that time was quietness and obedience.

So many of us have tried to do things our own way, which is probably what brought us to seeking a better way in the first place.

Just like Martha, we spent years manipulating diets, food, our bodies, our lives (and probably other people as well); being distracted, worried and upset that nothing "behaved itself" (or themselves), according to "our way"... getting so caught up in all the details that we missed the big picture!

Even when our motives are good, our methods might be wrong. Jesus did not tell Martha her preparations (works) were wrong, only her *consumption* with them – she was busy with the trees, while Mary was enjoying the forest!

Sometimes the only "work" Jesus requires of us is to sit humbly, willingly, patiently, obediently at His feet, just listening to what He has to say.

He wants us to just *"...be still and know that I am God."* (Psalms 46:10)

For some of us, though, that is the hardest thing of all. It is easier for us to be *"busy with preparations"* (doing "works" for God) than *"choosing what is better"* (learning of the "work" of God).

Dear Lord, help me to "see the forest through the trees," to choose what is better in Your sight, to not do things my way. Amen.

WEEK FOUR
DAY THREE

"Elisha replied to her, 'How can I help you? Tell me, what do you have in your house?' 'Your servant has nothing there at all,' she said, 'except a little oil.'"

How many of us feel ill-equipped to do what God has called us to do?

How often have we told the Holy Spirit, "Your servant has nothing here at all, except.." Except what? Except *obedience*! Except *willingness*! Except a *broken and contrite heart*! Except *faith* as small as a mustard seed! Yet if you have these things, *you have enough!*

This verse comes from a passage in 1Kings 4:1-7, about a widow whose creditors were coming to take her two sons as slaves. It shows us that God will use whatever you have, *no matter how little*, if you offer it willingly!

2Corinthians 8:12 says, *"For if the willingness is there, the gift is acceptable according to what one has, not according to what he does not have."*

Elisha told the widow to go around and ask all her neighbors for empty jars.

"Don't ask for just a few," he told her in verse 3.

Bringing them into her house, she filled them all with oil. The oil kept flowing until there were no jars left. Elisha then told the widow in verse 7, *"Go, sell the oil and pay your debts. You and your sons can live on what is left."*

How often we are content with settling for "just a few," when God wants to bless us abundantly!

What did the widow have, *"except a little oil,"* and yet, offered willingly to God, it was not only enough to meet the need, but enough to live on!

If you are struggling, questioning whether your meager resources are "enough" (whether financial or emotional), be encouraged by this passage. Your *obedience* and *willingness* are all God asks for. Then *He* will meet your needs.

Dear Lord, all I have is obedience and willingness, but what I do have, I offer to You. Please multiply my meager resources, as You did the widow's oil. Amen.

WEEK FOUR
DAY FOUR

"The Lord upholds all those who fall and lifts up all who are bowed down."

--Psa. 145:14

"It's me again, Lord...flat on my face. When will I learn to take it slow (or not at all)? Will I ever get it right? Will I ever be thin (again), or will I keep taking one step forward and two steps back? Will I ever taste the sweetness of victory instead of the bitter gall of defeat? I've tried this so many times before... what makes me think I can do it this time? I'm just not disciplined enough... I'm not good enough... I can't do it... I'm scared to try... I'm afraid to hope..."

Do any of these comments bring back memories to you? Or are any of them even recent thoughts?

Isn't it encouraging, then, to know that you're not alone? Whether in the area of food or any other bondage, the enemy has battled us in the way of these kinds of thoughts. Simply by using *fear* and *discouragement*, he can disarm us before we even set foot on the battlefield!

Yet if these were comments from someone you'd been witnessing to about salvation, what would you tell them?

Wouldn't you say that you don't have to "get it right," or "be good enough," or "be disciplined" to receive salvation... but that Jesus loves you just the way you are, and offers His gift freely and without conditions?

Victory in this area of our life is just as much a free gift as God's love, His gift of salvation. If you simply *receive* it, by grace, through no works of your own... just by obedience to His Word, responding to His love.

Isn't it encouraging to know that we're not doing this alone – that God is there... our loving gracious Lord who *"upholds all those who fall and lifts up all who are bowed down!"*

Dear Lord, I confess discouragement to You – I have felt like a failure so many times. But I take heart in Your Word, and believe in Your promise that You will give me victory in this area of my life. Thank You for upholding me and lifting me up. Amen.

WEEK FOUR
DAY FIVE

"Life is more than food, and the body more than clothes."

--Lk. 12:23

"Life is more than food?" What a novel idea!

I cringe as I recall all the years I spent scheduling my life around food... planning what to buy, what to cook, what to serve, what to eat... even church activities that all seemed attached to the words "pot luck dinner!"

Every major area of my life had food in it somewhere – high school graduation party, dinner dates, my wedding reception... even the chocolate basket my husband sent me after the birth of our son!

What a simple concept then, are the words *"life is more than food... "* reminding us that God had only meant food for sustenance of our bodies!

What a blessing it would be to be "God-centered" instead of "food-centered!"

To be re-centered on Christ, the "more" of our lives – to enter into sweet, loving fellowship with the One who centers Himself on us! Could we do anything less in return, than to focus ourselves back on the One who loves us most, and to return that love in joyful obedience?

Yes, praise God, life IS more than food!

John 14:6 says, *"Jesus answered, 'I am the way and the truth and the life. No one comes to the Father except through me." "I am the bread of life,"* Jesus said of Himself in John 6:48, and in John 6:51, He said, *"I am the living bread that came down from heaven. If anyone eats of this bread, he will live forever. This bread is my flesh, which I will give for the life of the world."*

Jesus IS our life, and the only "food" we really need!

Dear Lord, thank You for the life I have in You, and for re-focusing my eyes on my "living bread." Amen.

WEEK FOUR
DAY SIX

"Wait for the Lord; be strong and take heart and wait for the Lord."

--*Psa. 27:14*

"Be strong and take heart, all ye who hope in the Lord."

--*Psa. 31:24*

Patience was not exactly a virtue for me at one time; as I found myself tempted to "help God to help me" lose more weight. Instead of being content with the weight He'd already taken off me, I thought, "Well, if I just do this 'Cabbage Soup Diet' everyone at work is on, I'll lose the weight so much quicker, and God can then just *keep* it off me!"

What a lie! What seductive words from the devil! Praise God that in His "still small voice," He led me to the Psalms instead of the soup.

For some of us, our deepest testing comes in the area of *waiting* – waiting for God to work *His* perfect will in us, and not according to some agenda we have secretly set up for Him.

God says to *"be strong and take heart,"* knowing we will be tempted to do this the *quick* way, instead of the *permanent* way (in other words, *our* way, instead of *His* way).

God gives us these encouraging words in the Psalms, knowing how we would struggle. Even when we don't feel strong, our "taking heart" comes, again, by way of God's living Word, which gives us the hope that: *"I can do all things through Christ who gives me strength"* (Philippians 4:13), and knowing that: *"For when I am weak, then I am strong,"* through the strength of *Christ* (2Corinthians 12:10b).

Our hope in God comes from standing firm in His Word and on His promises, and in *waiting* for Him. Psalms 37:7 tells us to be still before the Lord and wait *patiently* for Him. We need to remember that God's timetable is not the same as ours, and while we're wanting to be thin "yesterday," the Lord looks at the bigger picture for us – that of the *character* He is building in us through this testing.

If we can learn the secret of waiting on the Lord, then we, like Abraham, will receive the blessings of obedience: *"And so after waiting patiently, Abraham received what was promised."* (Hebrews 6:15)

Dear Lord, help me to wait on You, to be patient as You work Your will in me, and to remember that I'd rather lose the weight permanently than to lose it quickly. Amen.

WEEK FOUR
DAY SEVEN

"Is not my house right with God? Has he not made with me an everlasting covenant, arranged and secured in every part? Will he not bring to fruition my salvation and grant me my every desire?"

--2Sam. 23:5

It's been said that the last words of a person's life are some of the most important ones. 2Samuel 23:1 begins with, *"These are the last words of David..."* and we see that in verse 5, we do read some of those last words.

What, then, was David most concerned about at that time? The same thing that most of us would be, also – whether his house was right with God.

What about you? Is your house right with God? Do you trust the everlasting covenant He has made with you? Do you believe that it has already been *"arranged and secured in every part?"*

Do you trust that God is true to His word – that He *will* bring to fruition *your* salvation? Even hope in Him enough to believe that He will grant you your *"every desire?"*

The God of David is *your* God today – He has never changed. What He did for David then, He can do for you today.

How did David know that his house was right with God? In Psalms 139:23, David had asked God to search his heart and test him, and in verse 24 said, *"See if there is any offensive way in me, and lead me in the way everlasting."* He was asking God to do some "housecleaning" in his heart and his life.

Could it be that God is using this time to do some "housecleaning" in your life, too? So that you, like David, can say, *"Is not my house right with God?"*

If so, submit to God – let Him search your heart and test you, and remove any way that is offensive in you – let Him gently and lovingly lead you in the way everlasting.

Dear Lord, please make my house right with You. Remove anything in my heart or in my life that is offensive to You, and lead me in the way everlasting. Amen.

WEEK FIVE
DAY ONE

"Set a guard over my mouth, O Lord; keep watch over the door of my lips. Let not my heart be drawn to what is evil, to take part in wicked deeds with men who are evildoers; let me not eat of their delicacies."

--Psa. 141:3-4

Willpower. Hah!

I have heard that some people actually do have willpower; alas, I am not one of them! Although a "successful dieter" in the past, lack of willpower sabotaged any permanent change in my eating habits.

Until God showed me how to lose weight *His* way, I equated the word "willpower" with "strength," and I knew I sure didn't have it!

Realizing that gluttony is a sin can be a real revelation to some of us. Just as I had felt that my willpower (or lack of it) had caused me to fall, and to again partake of "delicacies" I knew I shouldn't have, the Lord taught me that my mouth truly can lead me into sin.

What a wonderful God we serve, though, who even provides for my need to control my mouth!

Psalms 141:3-4 has become my prayer, just as important as the *"Lead me not into temptation, but deliver me from evil"* from the Lord's Prayer.

I know that I can't trust my own heart and mouth, which seem to be drawn more to "wicked deeds" than righteousness all too often. Yet God, in His faithfulness and desire to give us victory over food, has set this prayer before us as a *"way of escape."* (1Corinthians 10:13)

If you are struggling with when to stop eating, if you are not sure where "full" is yet, try saying these words out loud: *"Set a guard over my mouth, O Lord; keep watch over the door of my lips"* as your Grace before meals.

God will honor your desire, and keep you from the sin of gluttony.

Dear Lord, I thank You that I don't have to trust in my own willpower to save me from gluttony, but that You have already made provision for me in Your Word. Amen.

WEEK FIVE
DAY TWO

"But my eyes are fixed on you, O Sovereign Lord; in you I take refuge – do not give me over to death."

--Psa. 141:8

How many of us can fill in the blanks in the following: "Yes, Lord, I know that I've already lost ___ pounds, but I still have ___ pounds to go!"

It is a trick of the enemy to focus our eyes away from the success we've already achieved and toward anticipation of what is yet to be! This is contrary to God's Word, which says, *"Therefore do not worry about tomorrow, for tomorrow will worry about itself. Each day has enough trouble of its own."* (Matthew 6:34)

Matthew 6:33 says, *"But seek first his kingdom and his righteousness, and all these things will be given to you as well."* No wonder he can then follow with verse 34, which tells us to forget about tomorrow!

If we keep our eyes *fixed* on the Lord, take refuge in Him, and walk in obedience to Him *today*, tomorrow will take care of itself.

"One day at a time" has become such a popular saying because, in its simplicity, it is a very strong truth – we can't do anything about the past, and God says not to worry about tomorrow.

The only thing over which we have any control is *this* day, and whether we choose the way of obedience *today*.

In Luke 9:23, Jesus tells us that if we want to follow Him, we must deny ourselves and take up our cross *daily*. Joshua 24:15 says to choose *this* day whom you will serve.

Many of us become overwhelmed at how great the task appears before us, becoming discouraged at the mountain yet to climb. Yet, if we fix our eyes on the Lord, we will be reminded that *today* is all we really have to climb.

Dear Lord, help me to fix my eyes on You, and to remember that I can only do this "One day at a time," and then only with Your help. Amen.

WEEK FIVE
DAY THREE

"Then King David went in and sat before the Lord, and he said: 'Who am I, O Lord God, and what is my family, that you have brought me this far? And as if this were not enough in your sight, O God, you have spoken about the future of the house of your servant. You have looked on me as though I were the most exalted of men, O Lord God.'"

--1Chron. 17:16-17

It was so much easier for some of us to perceive ourselves as the "wretch" we sing of in the song, "Amazing Grace," than to accept ourselves as the *"royal priesthood"* of 1Peter 2:9.

Having struggled with being overweight most of my life, it was easy to agree with the world that I was a "wretch" who couldn't get her food problem under control.

But when I met Jesus, His loving eyes looked past my weight and into my heart, where He found a little girl longing to be loved. What a wonderful Savior, who looks past our appearances and through our hearts, all the way to our needs!

When a child has a fever, we can put him in a tub and try to cool him down from the outside in, or we can give him an aspirin to fix his fever from the inside out. "Dieting" was a way to fix me from the outside in, but not nearly as effective as when Jesus entered my heart and loved me (fixed me) from the inside out!

Isn't it encouraging to know that even King David struggled with being able to see himself as God saw him?

In 1Chronicles 17:16-17, he was basically asking God the same thing as we do – "Why would you notice *me*, Lord – and how can you look at me like I'm the most exalted of men, when I feel like I'm a wretch?"

How can He look at us that way? In the same way we can look at our children and see past their appearances and past their faults and failures, and love them with all our hearts from the inside out, as if they were *"the most exalted of men."*

Dear Lord, help me to see myself as You see me, and to accept Your unconditional love for me as love for myself. Amen.

WEEK FIVE
DAY FOUR

"But you are a chosen people, a royal priesthood, a holy nation, a people belonging to God, that you may declare the praises of him who called you out of darkness into his wonderful light."

--1Pet. 2:19

Some days I sure don't feel like a *"chosen people."* I sure wasn't very "royal" when the dishwater overflowed, and I didn't feel very "holy" when I yelled at my teenager... I sure can identify with the "darkness" of a gloomy day in which nothing seems to go right, though!

Even on the worst of days, we are still *"a people belonging to God;"* and no matter how dark the day may seem, with its myriad of things-gone-wrong, we are who we are so that we may *"declare the praises"* of a God who is more than able to deliver us from darkness!

Even when we don't *feel* like praising Him, as we draw closer to His light, our spirits will shed the darkness like an unwanted winter coat in the midst of a summer sun. As Christ begins to warm our hearts, we can do nothing else but praise Him!

Even Job, who had much more misfortune than we, said in Job 13:15, *"...though he slay me, yet will I hope in him."*

We can praise the Lord out of our *hope* in Him, like Job did. Like the old poster says, "Praise the Lord *anyway!*"

Nobody said it would be easy to praise the Lord in the midst of dirty tubs, dirty dishes, dirty houses and dirty children; but James 5:13 says, *"Is any one of you in trouble? He should pray. Is anyone happy? Let him sing songs of praise."*

The challenge, then, is to praise the Lord in the *midst* of the darkness, and to be happy as God brings us *out* of the darkness (dirtiness) of our lives.

Dear Lord, help me to praise You even when I don't feel like it. Even in the midst of darkness, let me dwell in Your wonderful light of deliverance. Amen.

WEEK FIVE
DAY FIVE

"Dear friends, I urge you, as aliens and strangers in the world, to abstain from sinful desires, which war against your soul."

--1Pet. 2:11

"O Lord, will I ever rise above the temptation of a Snickers bar?"

It was easy enough for me to associate my "sinful desires" with chocolate. Like many others in a meeting-based weight loss program, I couldn't stuff my face with it fast enough before that first meeting! Having been a "successful dieter" in the past, I knew that those candy bars would be the first thing to go, right? Wrong!

It is not chocolate, or any other food, in and of itself, that is sinful.

Romans 14:14 says, *"As one who is in the Lord Jesus, I am fully convinced that no food is unclean in itself. But if anyone regards something as unclean, then for him it is unclean."*

Food, then, isn't sin. It is the "sinful desire" in our hearts for the food, instead of for the Lord, that is wrong.

When I learned that "someday" I would be able to eat only half a candy bar and have no desire for the rest, my chocoholic mind screamed with laughter!

Yet, shortly into learning how to eat God's way, as I sought the Lord and His will for my eating habits... as I came into submission and obedience to His plan for my life... food (yes, even including chocolate) became less and less of a priority.

The day that I realized I'd actually *forgotten* about the candy bar in my purse for over a *week* was the day I realized that the Lord's sweet presence in my life was the only "chocolate" I really needed.

Dear Lord, I praise You for allowing the sweetness of Your presence in my life. Help me to keep You first, remembering that You are more important to me than any food. Amen.

WEEK FIVE
DAY SIX

"For the kingdom of God is not a matter of eating and drinking, but of righteousness, peace and joy in the Holy Spirit, because anyone who serves Christ in this way is pleasing to God and approved by men."

--Rom. 14:17-18

One of the main thrusts of this new way of eating is to help us to focus our hearts back to God, and get our priorities in order.

Many struggle with those first teachings of food as an *idol*, because it is difficult for us to see gluttony as a sin that has kept us from God. I mean, it's not like *adultery* or anything, right? Wrong!

In the eyes of God, sin is still sin. There is no sliding scale. *Anything* that comes between you and God is an idol, for then that thing is closer to God than you are! Nothing should come between you and God, not even food. When food has become your comforter, you have put it between you and God, *the* Comforter, the Holy Spirit.

Still questioning the sin of gluttony?

Then ask yourself if you have righteousness, peace and joy in the Holy Spirit. If you don't, then perhaps food *is* an idol in your life.

As Romans 14:17 teaches us, *"the kingdom of God is not a matter of eating and drinking..."*

Matthew 6:33 tells us to seek *first* the kingdom of God and *His* righteousness, and *then* our needs will be met.

It's a matter of priorities – let God be Lord over your whole life, including what you eat and drink, and you will watch the food idol topple and break into pieces.

When pleasing the Lord, and not your stomach, is the priority of your life, then righteousness, peace and joy will settle into your heart like a spring shower upon a dry flower.

Dear Lord, I repent of making food an idol – I don't want anything, especially food, to be closer to You than I am. Help me to keep my priorities straight, putting You before everything. Amen.

WEEK FIVE
DAY SEVEN

"Those who cling to worthless idols forfeit the grace that could be theirs."

--Jon. 2:8

How many of us laugh when Snoopy tries to take Linus' security blanket away from him, only to succeed in spinning Linus like a top, blanket intact? How many of us stop laughing, though, when the image becomes us, clinging so tightly to our security blanket of food that we end up spinning like a top as well?

Unfortunately, food has been very comforting to many of us – always there when we needed it, always enough (or, if not, we could always get more), always willing to listen and never give an opinion, something that never let us down.

Yet deep down, how many of us were truly satisfied with the comfort that food brought us?

A worthless idol is one that is empty, void, cold and unsatisfying; and isn't that, really, what food was to us? Sure, it never let us down, but it didn't lift us up, either.

Not like the *"friend who sticks closer than a brother"* of Proverbs 18:24, Jesus Christ.

God has given us a free will, but not without consequences; and there are always consequences for sin. We can choose to cling to food as a worthless idol, but what does Jonah 2:8 say that the consequences are? We will *forfeit* the grace that could be ours!

Romans 5:15 tells us, *"But the gift is not like the trespass. For if the many died by the trespass of the one man, how much more did God's grace and gift that came by the grace of the one man, Jesus Christ, overflow to many."*

Do we really want to forfeit this *grace* by clinging to a worthless idol? Not when God has so much more for us! In Romans 15:17 we are told, *"For if, by the trespass of the one man, death reigned through that one man, how much more will those who receive God's abundant provision of grace and of the gift of righteousness reign in life through the one man, Jesus Christ."*

Linus, let go of your blanket!

Dear Lord, help me to let go of food as my security blanket, and instead to cover myself with Your grace. Help me to accept the gift of Your grace. Amen.

WEEK SIX
DAY ONE

"Therefore, since we have been justified through faith, we have peace with God through our Lord Jesus Christ, through whom we have gained access by faith into this grace in which we now stand. And we rejoice in the hope of the glory of God."

--Rom. 5:1-2

Any successful 12-Step Program has, as its first step, the admission that the person is powerless over that which has held them in bondage.

The second step is to admit that only a Higher Power can deliver them from this bondage.

In Romans 5:1-2, we see this principle – nothing we can do on our own can deliver us from bondage; it is only by being *"justified through faith"* that we find peace with God, through Jesus and His grace.

Before learning to lose weight God's way, we were all standing on our own, trying in our own ways to find deliverance from food.

Yet this way points us back to Jesus, *"the author and finisher of our faith"* (Hebrews 12:2 KJV), because only through Jesus can we gain access, by faith, into His grace.

Only when we make Jesus Lord over us, can we truly stand – not on our own, but in His grace.

Is it any wonder, then, that when Jesus delivers us from the bondage of food, our entire countenance changes, and we walk around with smiles on our faces?

Deliverance is freedom, and freedom is joy, so that we can now *"rejoice in the hope of the glory of God."* (Romans 5:2)

Dear Lord, thank You for Your mercy, which delivers me from bondage and brings joy to my life. Amen.

WEEK SIX
DAY TWO

"No discipline seems pleasant at the time, but painful. Later on, however, it produces a harvest of righteousness and peace for those who have been trained by it."

--Heb. 12:11

Learning how to lose weight God's way, although not a "diet," does involve discipline.

Many of us failed in our attempts at man's way of losing weight because of a "lack of self-discipline."

Yet God's way is to teach us the discipline of obedience. We are to submit to God our Father, who will discipline us.

As He said in Hebrews 12:9, *"Moreover, we have all had human fathers who disciplined us and we respected them for it. How much more should we submit to the Father of our spirits and live!"*

Although the principles of eating God's way may seem simple at first, many of us find out very quickly that simple is not the same as easy. Just as Hebrews 12:11 tells us, *"no discipline seems pleasant at the time,"* discipline is not necessarily simple, easy, or pleasant.

Then why would a loving Heavenly Father want us to submit to something as unpleasant as discipline?

The answer is revealed in Romans 12:7, *"Endure hardship as disciple; God is treating you as sons. For what son is not disciplined by his father?"*

How many times have we told our own children, "I'm doing this for your own good?" So it is, then, that Romans 12:10 says, *"Our fathers disciplined us for a little while as they thought best; but God disciplines us for our good, that we may share in his holiness."* It is out of His great love for us that He leads us in the way of obedience.

Our Heavenly Father disciplines us because He loves us, so that this discipline would *"produce a harvest of righteousness and peace for those who have been trained by it."*

Dear Lord, help me to be obedient to Your discipline, to submit to it willingly, that I might Have that harvest of righteousness and peace. Amen.

WEEK SIX
DAY THREE

"My son, do not despise the Lord's discipline and do not resent his rebuke, because the Lord disciplines those he loves, as a father the son he delights in."

--Prov. 3:11-12

Submission… obedience… discipline…

Harsh words for those of us used to doing things our own way! How many of you picked up this book only to think it was just another set of rules to which you would adhere just until you lost the weight you wanted to lose, and then get on with your lives - only to find out that it isn't about "dieting" at all, but about obedience?

Somehow, in my rebellious "successful dieter's" heart, when God showed me how to lose weight *His* way, I was intimidated by the principles, because they seemed *too* easy for me.

"How will I know what to do?" I questioned at first, "What do You mean, just be obedient, Lord?" I questioned.

This was something new to me – something I couldn't control, and yet was given all this free-will control over! I had played God in the area of food in my life for so long that I wasn't too sure I wanted to give up the control, or accept this new way of control, either.

Yet God is so faithful, kind, and loving. *"Do not despise the Lord's discipline,"* He tells us. So it's not about "10 Steps to a Thinner Waistline," followed by a bunch of diet tips. It's about obedience to God, and *His* weight loss principles, as well as other areas of our lives.

"... and do not resent his rebuke," He goes on to say. Okay, so here I thought I was going to learn everything I was doing wrong in the way of dieting, but instead got some simple principles that even I could follow. The only rebuke I got was that I had been doing things *my* way and, instead, God wanted me to now do things *His* way.

Why does the Lord want it *His* way, the way of obedience and discipline? Because *"...the Lord disciplines those he loves, as a father the son he delights in."* Why? Because He *delights* in you! He loves you as your Father, and He *wants* you to succeed!

Dear Lord, thank You for loving me as a Father, and for disciplining me out of that love. Help me to be willing to submit to it. Amen.

WEEK SIX
DAY FOUR

"Let us fix our eyes on Jesus, the author and perfecter of our faith, who for the joy set before him endured the cross, scorning its shame, and sat down at the right hand of the throne of God. Consider him who endured such opposition from sinful men, so that you will not grow weary and lose heart."

--Heb. 12:2-3

Have you become discouraged lately – maybe not seen as many physical results of your obedience as you would have liked?

Have you been confronted by others who notice your weight loss has slowed down, or maybe even criticized your "non-diet" eating habits?

Discouragement sets in when we take our eyes off Jesus and again become self-centered or world-centered instead of Christ-centered.

The only way to *"...not grow weary and lose heart"* is to continually focus on Jesus, who died for you. He *"endured opposition from sinful men"* and *"endured the cross"* for the *joy* set before Him!

We, too, must endure our own crosses for the joy set before us, for the rewards of obedience.

If you focus on the opposition itself, it will draw your eyes away from the One who bore that opposition *for* you, so that you would *not* become weary and lose heart. He, Himself, then, is your encouragement.

Stand firm, then, in your obedience.

Fix your eyes on Jesus, and you will not only not grow weary, you will actually be *energized* by the joy you will receive from the Lord, for He gives us new joy each morning.

Dear Lord, help me to fix my eyes on You, and to receive the joy that comes from serving You with a whole heart. Amen.

WEEK SIX
DAY FIVE

"To the Jews who had believed him, Jesus said, 'If you hold to my teaching, you are really my disciples. Then you will know the truth, and the truth will set you free."

--Jn. 8:31-32

We so often concentrate on the unconditional love that Jesus had for us that we fail to see conditions on His teachings – I call it God's "If...Then's." Whenever you see these two words together (whether implied or stated) in the Word, take heed – it means that God requires something on your part.

Many times we hear John 8:32 quoted, without realizing that *before* we can know the truth, Jesus requires something on our part – it is only *if* we hold to His teachings that *then* we will know the truth, and the truth will set us free.

Sometimes the enemy comes against us and we feel as if we've been put "through the wringer" – especially if it's in an area in which we know we've been tested before, or even continually (like food); and we wonder if we'll *ever* have victory over this sin, or this area of testing. Yet, it is only when we can truly *hold* to the teachings of Christ that victory will come.

The only *offensive* weapon we have against the devil, according to Ephesians chapter 6, is the sword of the Spirit, which is the Word of God.

God is truth, and in Him there is no lie.

It is His Word that gives us victory, for in knowing the truth, we can stand against any temptation of the enemy – it is God's truth, in His Word, that truly does set us free.

And freedom… is victory!

Dear Lord, help me to stand firm and to not give up – to hold onto Your teachings so that I can stand strong against the enemy and would be delivered from bondage. Amen.

WEEK SIX
DAY SIX

"'No,' said Peter, 'you shall never wash my feet.' Jesus answered, 'Unless I wash you, you have no part with me.' 'Then, Lord,' Simon Peter replied, 'not just my feet but my hands and my head as well!'"

--Jn. 13:8-9

Have you been struggling in the area of obedience to God?

Are you walking in complete abandonment and total surrender to His will in your life, or are you still holding back that one part of your body you won't allow Jesus to wash?

Jesus told Peter, *"Unless I wash you, you have no part with me."*

Most of us have been more than willing to have Jesus have the weight problem in our lives. Yet for many of us, Jesus could not even get to the weight issue before first washing our *"hands and feet as well"* – before cleaning up the other areas of our lives in which we were not walking in obedience.

For some, it is easy to submit to these new principles, but very difficult to submit to, say, their spouse.

For others, it may be a struggle with their past, or their children, or personal faults, or a job situation, or any number of things.

Yet the Lord would have us submit *all* to Him, in order to deliver us out of *all* bondage. We must be willing to submit not just our weight problem to Him, but *every* area of our lives.

We must be filled with such total abandonment to Jesus that we cry out like Peter, *"Then, Lord, not just my feet but my hands and my head as well!"*

Dear Lord, I submit my life to You, and ask You to clean up any part of me that is not pleasing to You, so that I might walk in total obedience to You. Amen.

WEEK SIX
DAY SEVEN

"Cast your cares on the Lord and he will sustain you; he will never let the righteous fall."

--Psa. 56:22

I remember someone once telling me, "Be careful of your nevers – you always end up doing them!"

Some others have reminded me of the saying, "Never say never."

I know the old adage proved true in my own life, many times. "When *I* grow up," I muttered under my breath as a girl, "I'm *never* going to say to my children, 'Because I say so!'" I was *never* going to be like my parents, I swore – no way! Until I had my first child of course!

I was *never* going to fail – I was always going to succeed in life, no matter what I chose to do. Until I became an adult, of course, and lost my first job due to no fault of my own. It was then that I realized that it was necessary for me to redefine "success."

As a Christian, having gone through many trials and tribulations (as we all have), I realize what success really is, and how not to fail.

The answer lies in Psalms 56:22 – if you *"cast your cares on the Lord, and he will sustain you..."*

Our whole idea of success, our whole lives themselves, are redefined according to His perfect will for our lives!

God's "never" is the only "never" you never have to worry about!

He tells us in Psalms 55:2, *"I will never let the righteous fall,"* and in Hebrews 13:5, *"I will never leave you nor forsake you."*

How wonderful to know that we have such a loving, promise-keeping God, who "always" keeps his "nevers!"

Dear Lord, help me to trust in Your promises that You will never let me fail... that You will never leave me alone. Help me to cast my cares on You, so that You will sustain me. Amen.

WEEK SEVEN
DAY ONE

"Through him and for his name's sake, we received grace and apostleship to call people from among all the Gentiles to the obedience that comes from faith. And you also are among those who are called to belong to Jesus Christ."

--Rom. 1:5-6

The *obedience* that comes from faith... the obedience that comes *from faith*...

Knowing us in all our sin, knowing our shortcomings and failures, even knowing we would disappoint Him time and again, God still calls us to *"be among those who are called to belong to Jesus Christ"* – to be among those few chosen to learn this special obedience that comes from faith.

Are any of you from the "old school," where you learned obedience to your teacher by a ruler over your knuckles? Do you now remember the lesson being taught, or do you instead just remember the pain?

In Christ's school of obedience, the only ruler needed is the ruler of *love*.

Faith is not like a harsh wooden ruler across your hand – but, rather, like a butterfly that lights upon your shoulder... seemingly elusive sometimes, but when you have it, you are captivated by the beauty of its simplicity.

Perhaps that's why Jesus told us we must have faith as a child - so that we would not complicate this thing. And, as adults, isn't that what we do try to do with this "obedience-thing?"

Hebrews 11:1 says, *"Now faith is being sure of what we hope for and certain of what we do not see."*

Following man-made rules and diets, many of us were able to manipulate our way through weight loss. Yet it is *this* kind of faith, the kind talked about in Hebrews, through which the Lord would have you learn *"the obedience that comes from faith."*

Dear Lord, teach me the obedience that comes from faith so that my body, mind, and spirit might come into line with Your good and perfect will for me. Amen.

WEEK SEVEN
DAY TWO

"Then he said to Thomas, 'Put your finger here, see my hands. Reach out your hand and put it into my side. Stop doubting and believe.' Thomas said to him, 'My Lord and my God!' Then Jesus told him, 'Because you have seen me, you have believed; blessed are those who have not seen and yet have believed."

--Jn. 20:27-29

How many of us have already seen a vision, or have a mental picture of what we will look like when we've lost the weight we want to lose?

Then how many of us get discouraged because we have yet to see the physical evidence of that inner work?

Like Thomas, we sometimes feel the need to actually touch something before we believe it is real. Yet that is the world's way and *not* God's way!

How many of us used scales (physical evidence, something we could touch) to determine our weight loss success before learning these new principles? Now how many of us have forsaken the scales to begin our "trust-walk" in the Lord to show us evidence of our weight loss *His* way?

Hasn't God been faithful in the past? Has He not always done what He has promised?

In our own lives, can't we all list many times that we *know* the Lord had His hand in some event or miracle in our lives? We've put our fingers on Him – we've had our hand in His side – we have seen Him as evidenced all around us! Then why would we doubt Him in this thing?

Jesus commands us to *"Stop doubting and believe."* Recall the work He's already done in your life, and *trust* Him to finish the work He has started now in you.

If faith is *"being sure of what we hope for and certain of what we do not see,"* as Hebrews 11:1 tells us it is, then we can all trust in our minds-eye picture of ourselves, even though we may not have physical evidence of it yet. Then we, too, can be among those who are blessed because we *"have not seen and yet have believed."*

Dear Lord, thank You for the vision You have given me. Help me to trust in You to bring it to pass. Give me the faith to believe in Your promise, even without physical evidence. Amen.

WEEK SEVEN
DAY THREE

"Early in the morning, Jesus stood on the shore, but the disciples did not realize that it was Jesus. He called out to them, 'Friends, haven't you any fish?' 'No,' they answered. He said, 'Throw your net on the right side of the boat and you will find some.' When they did, they were unable to haul the net in because of the large number of fish."

--Jn. 21:4-6

Are you still struggling with the idea that Jesus is interested in your weight loss?

Do you not yet trust that God is concerned about you (Exodus 4:3) and will perfect *all* that concerns you (Psalms 138:8 KJV)?

Are you like the disciples on the shore, who did not realize it was Jesus?

Could it be that you "haven't any fish" (any physical evidence of weight loss) because your net is still tossed on the wrong side of the boat? Are you still trying to walk God's plan for you... *your way*?

Listen to your Lord, who loves you and wants the best for you... listen to *"him who is able to do immeasurably more than all we ask or imagine, according to his power that is at work within us"* (Ephesians 3:20), and let Him have His way in you.

Stop struggling to fish on your own.

111

Realize that this truly is Jesus, and cast your net on the right side of the boat, as He commands.

Then you, like the disciples, will find that God's way *does* meet your needs, and abundantly so!

Dear Lord, I believe that You are concerned for me, and that You want only the best for me. Help me to listen to You and to stop struggling with trying to do things my own way. Amen.

WEEK SEVEN
DAY FOUR

"Moses and Aaron brought together all the elders of the Israelites, and Aaron told them everything the Lord had said to Moses. He also performed the signs before the people, and they believed. And when they heard that the Lord was concerned about them and had seen their misery, they bowed down and worshiped."

--Exod. 4:29-31

All of our lives have been touched by the Lord, or we wouldn't be here today. Like the Israelites, we all need to be reminded sometimes of how far we have actually come... of everything the Lord has said to us... of everything he has done for us.

Signs have also been performed for/by many of us, and we have believed.

Have you been feeling alone in your struggle lately? Have you been unable to feel God's touch in this?

Then may you again be reminded now that your Lord truly is concerned about you. He has seen your misery. There is nothing that escapes God's sight.

If He is concerned about the birds of the air (Luke 12:24) and the grass of the field (Luke 12:27), how much more is He concerned for you? He says not to be afraid, *"for your Father has been pleased to give you the kingdom."* (Luke 12:32)

What parent does not want the best for their child? As Luke 11:11-13 says, *"Which of you fathers, if your son asks for a fish, will give him a snake instead? Or if he asks for an egg, will give him a scorpion? If you then, though you are evil, know how to give good gifts to your children, how much more will your Father in heaven give the Holy Spirit to those who ask him!"*

Ask He who is the Lord of the harvest (Matthew 9:38) to plant His seed in you.

Ask Him to send you His Holy Spirit, the Comforter, who will guide you in all your ways (John 14:26). And you will never be alone again, as you, like the Israelites, bow down and worship your God.

Dear Lord, You are my Heavenly Father, who is concerned for me, and I believe You have seen my misery. I bow down and worship You, my Father and my God. Amen.

WEEK SEVEN
DAY FIVE

"On the last and greatest day of the Feast, Jesus stood and said in a loud voice, 'If anyone is thirsty, let him come to me and drink. Whoever believes in me as the Scripture has said, streams of living water will flow from within him.' By this he meant the Spirit, whom those who believed in him were later to receive. Up to that time the Spirit had not been given, since Jesus had not yet been glorified."

--Jn. 7:37-39

Has your walk in this desert of testing been a dry one?

Are you thirsty for the "living water" that should be flowing through you?

Could it be that you have been busily learning *about* the water, instead of just accepting it as a *gift?*

Jesus told the woman at the well, *"If you knew the gift of God and who it is that asks you for a drink, you would have asked him and he would have given you living water."* (John 4:10) *"...Whoever drinks the water I give him will never thirst. Indeed, the water I give him will become in him a spring of water welling up to eternal life!"* (John 4:14)

Like the woman at the well, if you are thirsty in this hot, dry, lonely desert of testing, you need only to ask, *"Sir, give me this water..."* (John 4:15a)

This water, according to John 7:39, is the Holy Spirit. At that time, Jesus had not yet been glorified, so the people had not been given the Spirit – but this day the Lord *has* been glorified, and the gift of God is eternal life through Jesus Christ His Son!

This gift is given freely to all who would ask. To all who would call upon His name, the gift of salvation is given freely.

To those who have already received the gift of salvation, another gift is offered – the gift of the Holy Spirit.

Jesus said, *"If you love me, you will obey what I command. And I will ask the Father, and he will give you another Counselor to be with you forever..."* (John 14:15-16)

Dear Lord, thank You for the gift of my salvation. I ask You now for the gift of the Holy Spirit, the Counselor, who will be with me forever. Amen.

WEEK SEVEN
DAY SIX

"So I say to you: Ask and it will be given to you; seek and you will find; knock and the door will be opened to you. For everyone who asks receives; he who seeks finds and to him who knocks, the door will be opened."

--Lk. 11:9-10

Some of you may have been "walking this walk" for quite awhile now – many have been Christians for a long time.

So maybe even before you found this book and began this desert of testing, you were already experiencing a desert in your own spiritual walk.

All of us experience a "dry" time spiritually – a time of walking through the valley. Our spiritual walk cannot consist solely of mountaintop experiences; for as wonderful as it is on the Mountain of the Lord, it is in the valley where we learn God's deepest secrets.

It is the lessons learned in the desert of testing that conform us into the image of Christ. If He endured the desert, could we do any less?

Yet many question their salvation when walking in the valley, and/or want to leave the valley.

But Jesus commanded the disciples *not* to leave Jerusalem (in other words, to stay in their "valley"), but to wait – *"...wait for the gift my Father promised, which you have heard me speak about. For John* baptized with water, but in a few days you will be baptized with the Holy Spirit." (Acts 1:4-5)

Or you might believe in your salvation, but question the *power* of it.

Jesus said in Acts 1:8, *"But you will receive power when the Holy Spirit comes on you..."*

Could it be that although you are saved, you have yet to receive the Holy Spirit? Could it be that today is *your* "Day of Pentecost?" (Acts 1 and 2)

You have only to "ask, seek, and knock," according to Luke 11:9, *"...and you will receive the gift of the Holy Spirit."* (Acts 2:38)

Dear Lord, I believe in Your Word. I believe in my salvation. Now let me believe in the Holy Spirit, whom You have sent. Let me receive this power from on high. Amen.

WEEK SEVEN
DAY SEVEN

"Now, Lord, consider their threats and enable your servants to speak your word with great boldness. Stretch out your hand to heal and perform miraculous signs and wonders through the name of your holy servant Jesus."

--Acts 4:29-30

"After they prayed, the place where they were meeting was shaken. And they were all filled with the Holy Spirit and spoke the word of God boldly."

--Acts 4:31

Have you ever wondered why you were "singled out" by God for this testing? And even when you have felt like a Job in your struggles, have you harbored in your heart the knowledge that you have not been doing this for yourself alone?

When you received salvation, was it not a fire that burned so brightly within you that you wanted to give it away to the whole world? And yet have you, over the years, felt like you've lost your joy?

David, the wonderful Psalmist, the great king, felt that way, too! He asked God in Psalms 51:12, *"Restore to me the joy of your salvation and grant me a willing spirit to sustain me."*

With but a willing spirit, you can again experience the joy of the Lord; you can willingly pray the disciples' prayer of Acts 4:29-30 (above). Then *your* mountain, too, will be shaken, and you will be

119

filled with the Holy Spirit, speaking the word of God boldly (Acts 4:31).

Then you will know that you have not done this for yourself alone – but for the others you will touch by your testimony. When you speak God's Word with boldness, signs and wonders will be performed through the name of Jesus. And Jesus said you would do even greater things than the disciples did (John 14:12)!

This has not been for yourself alone: *"The promise is for you and your children and for all who are far off – for all whom the Lord our God will call."* (Acts 2:39)

Dear Lord, I thank You and praise You for the work You have done in me. Thank You for the gift of the Holy Spirit. Help me now to speak Your Word boldly, as I tell others of Your love and Your gifts. Amen.

WEEK EIGHT
DAY ONE

"But nothing that a man owns and devotes to the Lord – whether man or animal or family land – may be sold or redeemed; everything so devoted is most holy to the Lord."

--Lev. 27:28

How many times do we give something to the Lord, only to take it back again?

And isn't it usually because either God didn't do what we asked, or that He didn't do it our way, or that He didn't do it fast enough?

The Hebrew term for "devotes" in Leviticus 27:28 refers to the *irrevocable giving over* of things or persons to the Lord.

Webster's dictionary defines "irrevocable" as "incapable of being recalled;" that is, it cannot be taken back. For some of us, the issue is not in the "giving over," it is in the "not taking back!"

We must learn to *devote* to God, give to the Lord, without ever expecting anything in return, and without ever trying to take it back.

Whether it is our desires, hopes and dreams... or whether it is our children, our marriages, our jobs, our futures... or whether it is the results we hope to achieve by learning to eat God's way... we can only *devote* it (them) to the Lord and *trust* Him for the results.

When we take something (or someone) to the altar and lay our burden at the feet of our Lord, we must walk away with a conviction to leave it (them) there, trusting that the Lord is big enough to handle it... and that He's capable enough to handle it *without our help!*

Only in this way will our "sacrifice of devotion," our *"everything so devoted,"* truly be *"most holy to the Lord."*

Dear Lord, help me to trust You with all my cares, devoting them to Your loving care, and leaving them there at Your altar. Help me, Lord, not to try to "help" You, but to trust the results to You, not trying to take anything back. Amen.

WEEK EIGHT
DAY TWO

"Immediately he spoke to them and said, 'Take courage! It is I. Do not be afraid.' He climbed into the boat with them, and the wind died down."

--Mk. 6:50-51

Mark 6:51 is the last line of a familiar passage of Scripture (Mark 6:45-51), where Jesus walks on the water.

A storm had arisen, and the disciples, alone in a boat tossing about the raging waters, were afraid.

We are told in Mark 6:46 that Jesus had gone up on a mountainside to pray – yet we see that He never took His eyes off His disciples!

We know this, because of Mark 6:48, where we read, *"He saw the disciples straining at the oars, because the wind was against them."*

What did Jesus do? According to Mark 6:48, *"he went out to them."*

What did the disciples do? They cried out in terror!

Why did the disciples cry out in terror, when this was their own Jesus coming out to them? Because they were so afraid that they didn't even recognize Him as Jesus!

How many times are we so overwhelmed by the wind against us that we fail to recognize Jesus in the midst of *our* own struggle?

Jesus did two things then: According to Mark 6:50-51, *"Immediately he spoke to them and said, 'Take courage! It is I. Do not be afraid.' He climbed into the boat with them, and the wind died down."* He not only *spoke* to them in their "storm," but also *joined* them in it!

In the midst of your struggle, whatever the wind be against you, hearken to the words of Jesus – do not be afraid, and let Him climb into your boat with you. He will calm the wind in *your* life.

Dear Lord, just like the disciples, I am so often terrified of the wind and storms against me. Help me to recognize You in this, and to know that You will calm the winds for me. Amen.

WEEK EIGHT
DAY THREE

"Then the Lord answered Job out of the storm."
                                                    --Job 38:1
"Then the Lord spoke to Job out of the storm."
                                                    --Job 40:6

Notice that it doesn't say "before the storm" (to warn Job of it)... or "after the storm" (that He wasn't there during it)... not "when the storm was quiet" (so that Job could hear Him louder)... but *"out of the storm"* – in the *midst* of it, while it still raged about Job.

If we were to wait to only hear from God when it is peaceful and quiet, we might never hear from God at all!

Or if we expect Him to speak before a storm, warning us of impending disaster, we will be disappointed when He doesn't do it.

Or if we ask the Lord, "Where were you?" after the storm has passed, we might realize that we had already missed Him.

BUT... if we will be quiet in the *midst* of our storms... if we will seek His presence while the storm still rages all about us... God might very well speak to us *"out of the storm,"* as He did to Job.

Some of us are afraid that God doesn't *see* our storms... we feel all alone in the struggles confronting us. But Job says in Job 31:4, *"Does he not see my ways and count my every step?"*

And doesn't God say in Deuteronomy 31:6 to: *"Be strong and courageous. Do not be afraid or terrified because of them, for the Lord your God goes with you; he will never leave you or forsake you."*

And again in verse 8, *"The Lord himself goes before you and will be with you; he will never leave you nor forsake you. Do not be afraid; do not be discouraged."*

Take heart, whatever your "storms," that your Heavenly Father knows who you are, where you are, and what your struggles are.

Dear Lord, thank You for Your Word, reminding me that You will never leave me nor forsake me, and that You are with me in the midst of my storms. Amen.

WEEK EIGHT
DAY FOUR

"Jesus left that place and went to the vicinity of Tyre. He entered a house and did not want anyone to know it; yet he could not keep his presence secret."

--Mk. 7:24

What was it about Jesus that He could not keep His presence secret upon entering a house?

Could it be the *"glory of the Lord"* referred to in Scriptures, that shown about His face? Could it be the presence of the Holy Spirit, reflected in the countenance of Jesus? Could it be the very air about Him, that carried with it the presence of God the Father?

What about you? Do you so reflect the presence of Jesus that He cannot *"keep his presence secret?"* Or do you too often hear those condemning words, "Oh, I didn't know you were a Christian!"

Jesus commands us in Matthew 5:16, *"Let your light so shine before men, that they may see your good works, and glorify your Father which is in heaven."*

The Lord does not want us to hide our joy, to hide our hope of glory, which is in Christ Jesus – in fact, he wants us to spread *"the fragrance of him"* everywhere we walk!

Our daily walk with Jesus should be so active with His presence that we could no more keep Him a secret than He Himself could, when he entered that house. Our outward appearance must reflect the inner presence of a Holy God.

Jesus said in Luke 12:8, *"Whoever confesses me before men"* (i.e., confesses his love by everything he does, not merely by words or deeds), *"him the Son of Man also will confess before the angels of God."*

Don't be condemned by the words, "Oh, I didn't know you were a Christian!"

Let your very presence in a room be so filled with the presence of the Holy Spirit, that your light will shine brightly, no matter how dark the room.

Dear Lord, help me to be more like You. Let me be so full of Your presence, that everyone will know that You are my Lord. Amen.

WEEK EIGHT
DAY FIVE

"What other nation is so great as to have their gods near them the way the Lord our God is near us whenever we pray to him?"

--Deut. 4:7

When the Presidential Primaries were going on, I had to pause and consider how much we take for granted the freedoms of our great nation.

Back in the book of Deuteronomy, it seemed, they asked themselves the same question.

How fortunate we are to be able to pray, and how sad to think that we take this freedom for granted!

We hear about other religions, even cults, who claim to have the "real" God; yet, we sometimes hide the fact that we DO have the one real, true, *living* God, whose very presence is active in our lives... who listens to our concerns... who responds to our prayers!

What greater privilege can there be than the "privilege of prayer?"

Whether our struggle is with food or any other bondage, the principle of obedience taught in the Scriptures is the only deliverance unto *true freedom!*

Because this kind of obedience can only be learned through total and complete submission to our

Lord Jesus Christ, the only one able to deliver us from our sins.

How can we experience this deliverance?

By drawing near to the God who *"is near us whenever we pray to him."*

Draw near to God, and He will draw near to you.

Dear Lord, as I pray to You, as I draw near to You, I ask that You draw near to me, for I need Your holy presence in my life today. Amen.

WEEK EIGHT
DAY SIX

"Therefore I tell you, whatever you ask for in prayer, believe that you have received it, and it will be yours."

--Mk. 11:24

Many times we find conditions to obtaining our desires in God's Word (remember my "If...Then's?").

For instance, in the passage just before this one, Jesus says (verse 23), *"I tell you the truth, if anyone says to this mountain, 'Go, throw yourself into the sea,' and does not doubt in his heart but believes that what he says will happen, it will be done for him."*

Note that He says *if* he says...and *does not doubt... [then]* it will be done for him.

God is faithful to His promises, like He says in Mark 11:24, but sometimes He expects us, through our own choices and actions, to do something in order to receive.

What, then, is there for us to do to receive these promises, these answers to prayer?

We need to: (1) pray, (2) not doubt, (3) believe, and then (4) receive (sometimes the hardest thing to do).

How can we do all this? Look back at verse 22 of this passage, and there is your answer: *"'Have faith in God,' Jesus answered."*

In verse 24, it seems, all you have to do is believe you have already received it, and you will.

Ah, but don't we tend to say to ourselves, "That's too simple!" And then don't we set about immediately to complicate it?

But faith *is* a simple thing. We need only to *"Have faith in God,"* believing Him to be willing and able to answer our prayers.

Dear Lord, help me to believe, and not doubt, that You will answer my prayers. Increase my faith, so that I will believe the mountains confronting me <u>will</u> move. Amen.

WEEK EIGHT
DAY SEVEN

"Be careful to obey all these regulations I am giving you, so that it may always go well with you and your children after you, because you will be doing what is good and right in the eyes of the Lord your God."

--Deut. 12:28

Have you ever wondered why, so many times in the Old Testament (especially in Leviticus and Deuteronomy, where Moses is listing out all the laws), you read the words, *"...so that it may go well with you and your children after you?"*

Consider this – your children are watching every move that you make. You are their example.

If you are rebellious and disobedient, that is what will be passed down generation to generation (like the people of Israel).

On the other hand, *"...if you do what is good and right in the eyes of the Lord your God,"* your children will see this and imitate it, and it *will* go well for them.

Children imitate what they see. That is how they learn, and that is how they live.

That's why in Ephesians 5:1, Paul says, *"Be imitators of God, therefore, as dearly loved children..."*

Be careful, then, how you live your life before your children, for your children are watching you.

Other people are watching you, too. Have you noticed stares from other people, even received comments, as others have noticed your weight loss?

Let God use this as an opportunity to "be a testimony" to His power working in your life, as you submit, in obedience, to His will for you.

In this way, you *will* be doing *"...what is good and right in the eyes of the Lord your God."*

Dear Lord, help me to live a righteous life before my children, that they might also know the righteousness of Christ. Let me be a witness to others of Your power working in my life. Amen.

WEEK NINE
DAY ONE

"Some women were watching from a distance. Among them were Mary Magdalene, Mary the mother of James the younger and Joses, and Salome. In Galilee these women had followed him and cared for his needs. Many other women who had come up with him to Jerusalem were also there."

--Mk. 15:40-41

We hear so much talk about the "modern woman" – who she is, what great things she's accomplished… We hear about her in a worldly way, though – her success is measured by worldly standards.

Why, the "modern woman," (a perfect size 5, of course) is the perfect wife and homemaker, perfect PTA Mom while balancing family and job responsibilities at the same time, leader of her circle of friends; she is always everything to everybody!

Right. And how many of *us* fit that model? Of course it's impossible, because God never designed us to be that way.

He made woman *separate* from man, unique in her own right, but as a helpmeet for man – to serve her husband and family, but not to "run the whole show!" And especially not perfectly, at that.

God never meant for a woman to be judged by her accomplishments, nor by her outward appearance (as the world does), but by her *heart.*

God's Word tells us in Proverbs 31:30, *"Charm is deceptive, and beauty is fleeting; but a woman who fears the Lord is to be praised."*

Whether it is the 1500's or 2000's, God's design for a woman has never changed. Like the two Mary's in Mark 15:40-41, we are to *follow Jesus* and *care for His needs.*

What needs of Jesus is He calling you to meet? Are you to be His hands in caring for the children? His voice to a dying generation? To anoint His presence with oil? Or, simply, to pray?

Whatever He has called you to do, He needs you to do it.

Dear Lord, help me to be faithful to meet Your needs today. Let me be like the two Mary's, looking to meet Your needs before my own. Amen.

WEEK NINE
DAY TWO

"And that you may love the Lord your God, listen to his voice, and hold fast to him. For the Lord is your life..."

--Deut. 30:20

President John F. Kennedy once said, "Ask not what your country can do for you; ask what you can do for your country."

One of his best-known quotes, he was calling for a unified, patriotic nation whose eyes were turned away from their own selfish needs, and toward the greater good; that of serving their country.

Well, I would challenge you this day with these words: "Ask not what your Lord can do for you; ask what you can do for your Lord."

Not as well-known a quote, perhaps, but just as sincere and probing in its challenge for you to turn away from your selfish needs, and toward the greater good; that of serving your Master.

What does the Lord require of you?

According to Luke 10:27, it is that, *"You shall love the Lord your God with all your heart, with all your soul, with all your strength, and with all your mind, and your neighbor as yourself."*

You are to love Him, to listen to His voice, and to hold fast to Him, for the Lord truly *is* your life. If you do this first (and always), you will then be able to love others and yourself.

We are in the "Lord's army," called to give our lives in service for the King.

We must ask ourselves, as soldiers of the Lord, how we can serve Him best. Then, as good soldiers, we must walk in courage and servitude.

Dear Lord, help me to love You better, hear You louder, hold fast to You tighter, and to serve You with my whole heart, soul, strength, and mind. Amen.

WEEK NINE
DAY THREE

"Teach me your way, O Lord, and I will walk in your truth; give me an undivided heart, that I may fear your name."

--Psa. 87:11

One day, my four sons came to me and challenged me with the question, "Mommy, which one of us do you love the most?"

Not satisfied with my quick answer of, "Well, I love all of you the same," they continued, "Yes but who the *most*?"

I answered them, "I love Travis the most because I did not give birth to him; he was a gift to me when he was five years old. I love Kerry the most, because he was my firstborn child. I love CJ the most because he is so unique and creative, and I love Tyler the most because he is my baby."

This, of course, stunned them into thought; however, shortly their cries rang out again, "But Mom..."

I simply smiled at my beloved sons. How could I explain to them that it was just impossible to divide my heart that way?

Fear of the Lord is an awesome, reverent love for Him. This kind of love must be served from an undivided heart.

For that is the kind of heart our Heavenly Father has for *His* children, and He could no more divide His heart toward us, than I could divide mine toward my children!

Ours is a jealous God, who wants us to have an undivided heart toward Him, like His toward us. How, then, can we continue to divide our hearts between God and food?

Matthew 6:24 says, *"No one can serve two masters. Either he will hate the one and love the other, or he will be devoted to the one and despise the other. You cannot serve both God and money."*

In the same way I challenge you: You cannot love (serve) both God and food.

Dear Lord, give me an undivided heart toward You, that I may fear Your name. Let me learn to accept Your undivided heart toward me. Amen.

WEEK NINE
DAY FOUR

"I love them that love me; and those that seek me early shall find me."

--Prov. 8:17 KJV

Many of us have a devotional time set aside in the morning; many agree that seeking the Lord first thing seems to "start their day" much better. I have even heard it referred to as "tithing the first 10% of your day."

Whether you have a morning devotion or an evening devotion, the most important thing is that you do seek Him; that you do spend time with the Lord.

The NIV version of the Bible uses the word "earnestly" instead of "early." More importantly than the time of day you choose to seek the Lord is how *earnestly* you seek Him, and the quality of time you spend with Him.

Compare a morning devotion (for the Spirit) to a breakfast meal (for the body).

It would be foolish to assume that one bowl of oatmeal would be enough to sustain your body throughout the entire day without replenishing the nourishment your body craves.

In the same way, it is foolish to assume that one small dose of Jesus in the morning would be enough spiritual nourishment to carry you through an entire day!

We must all seek the Lord "earnestly," throughout our days; to seek the Lord at every opportunity as the day progresses. 1Thessalonians 5:17 tells us to *"pray continually."*

We feed our bodies periodically throughout our days; why not feed our spirits as well? We certainly don't expect that one breakfast meal to sustain us the entire day. How then can we submit to less for our spiritual bodies?

We begin each day with a certain amount of energy for that day, both physical and spiritual. Taking time to "recharge" that energy at times during the day is healthy for body *and* spirit.

Dear Lord, let me not be too busy to take time out for You during my day. Sustain me with Your Word and Your presence throughout my busy days. Amen.

WEEK NINE
DAY FIVE

"How priceless is your unfailing love! Both high and low among men find refuge in the shadow of your wings. They feast on the abundance of your house; you give them drink from your river of delights."

--Psa. 36:7-8

How often have we settled for "second best?" For an artificial love, or a conditional love; even a counterfeit love?

How often have people even tried to *buy* this "second best" love?

Yet we have a wonderful Heavenly Father who offers us an *unfailing* love, and David says in Psalms 36 that this unfailing love is *priceless!*

It is this love, this priceless, unfailing love, with which God surrounds us when we find refuge in the shadow of His wings; when we abide in Him.

How often have we settled for "second best" when it comes to food as well?

We have settled for an artificial pleasure; a conditional pleasure; even a counterfeit pleasure. How many of us have found this type of pleasure unsatisfactory! Well you did, or you wouldn't be reading this book!

Yet our Heavenly Father, who trades ashes for riches, life for death, sinfulness for righteousness... longs to trade our "second best" pleasure for the *absolute* best He has to offer!

If we are willing to trade in our counterfeit food idol, He promises us that we can feast on the abundance of *His* house. He will give us drink from *His* river of delights!

How priceless is this type of living in the refuge of a Heavenly Father who offers us only the best – *His* best.

Dear Lord, help me to release my food idol to You, gladly receiving in return the abundance of all the riches You have in store for me. Amen.

WEEK NINE
DAY SIX

"Then the word of the Lord came to Jeremiah; 'I am the Lord, the God of all mankind. Is anything too hard for me?'"

--Jer. 32:26-27

Have you been limiting God? Have you been lowering Him to your standards, instead of raising yourself up to His? Have you been trying to make Him conform to some earthly fatherly image you have set Him up to be, instead of getting to know Him as the Heavenly Father which He is?

In our own insecurity, we stumble around blindly trying to find our own way, limited by our small understanding of the circumstances confronting us, without considering what God says in Isaiah 55:9, *"As the heavens are higher than the earth, so are my ways higher than your ways and my thoughts higher than your thoughts."*

Many times we are like the Israelites in the desert – wandering helplessly, concerned only for the meeting of our immediate physical needs. Yet the Lord tells us to keep our eyes on Him, and *not* on the circumstances surrounding us.

1Corinthians 13:12 talks about seeing *"a poor reflection as in a mirror"* (in KJV as seeing *"through a glass darkly"*). We cannot trust our own perception of our circumstances.

We cannot limit God to our own way of thinking – we need to trust Him to bring His plans into being, His way. We not only need to forsake our way of doing things, but also to forsake our limited understanding of God's way of doing things.

We need to abandon ourselves so totally to Christ that His way *becomes* our ways; so that, instead of lowering Him to our level, we are raised to His.

Do you still limit God? Or can you now believe in His "higher ways;" His limitless ability to deliver you from your bondage?

Is anything too hard for God? No! *"Ah, Sovereign Lord, you have made the heavens and the earth by your great power and outstretched arm. Nothing is too hard for you."* (Jeremiah 32:17)

Dear Lord, I trust in Your unfailing love. I know Your ways are higher than mine, and I do believe that nothing is too hard for You. Please, dear Lord, deliver me from this bondage. Amen.

WEEK NINE
DAY SEVEN

"This is what the Lord says: 'Maintain justice and do what is right, for my salvation is close at hand and my righteousness will soon be revealed. Blessed is the man who does this, the man who holds it fast, who keeps the Sabbath without desecrating it, and keeps his hand from doing any evil."

--Isa. 56:1-2

For a country built on freedom, we sure seem to have a lot of rules, don't we?

Even in the Bible – it took whole books to contain all the laws! Sometime we might ask ourselves if there aren't too many laws... or if the laws are just... or even why we need to obey all these rules and laws?

In our society, the advantage of keeping the laws is simply to avoid being arrested and put in jail. Yet God's laws are different – they don't come with a threat, they come with a *promise!*

God promises that if we keep *His* laws, we will receive blessings. If we *"maintain justice and do what is right,"* God will bring His salvation close and His *"righteousness will soon be revealed."*

Although there are not any man-made laws in God's way of eating healthy, there are some "rules," or principles, we are asked to follow. Some of you may question these "rules," asking: Are they valid? Do I need to follow them? Why should I submit to them? Because your way didn't work, and God's way does work, that's why!

Some people (out of rebellion), choose not to follow these rules. Okay, so you won't be arrested for breaking the law, but couldn't you also be missing out on the blessings that God has in store for you?

If you will submit to the rules as outlined in the beginning of this book, as well as to God's law, you will soon see His righteousness revealed in you. You will be allowing His salvation to deliver you from bondage.

"Blessed is the man who does this, the man who holds it fast..." If you "keep on keeping on," obeying God's laws and keeping your hand from doing evil, you will experience the salvation of God close at hand, and you will truly be blessed.

Dear Lord, I again confess my rebellion to You. Help me to obey Your laws, and to hold fast to Your principles, that Your righteousness would be revealed in me. Amen.

WEEK TEN
DAY ONE

"As the rain and snow come down from heaven, and do not return to it without watering the earth and making it bud and flourish, so that it yields seed for the sower and bread for the eater, so is my word that goes out from my mouth: It will not return to me empty, but will accomplish what I desire and achieve the purpose for which I sent it."

--Isa. 55:10-11

We trust in things we can see with our own eyes – it is easy to believe in the rain and the snow, because we can see them come down.

We can even trust in the results of that rain, because we see the flowers bud and the plants flourish.

We gratefully partake of the food of the earth, having watched it grow and often having even harvested it ourselves.

So we believe in the whole process, because we have seen it and touched it.

How much more difficult it is for us, though, to believe in God's Word accomplishing the same thing spiritually that His rain does physically.

Jesus told Thomas in John 20:29, *"Because you have seen me you have believed; blessed are those who have not seen and yet have believed."*

God's Word is His promise.

He has promised each of us that His Word, if planted in us, will accomplish what He desires and achieve His purposes for us.

God has a plan for each one of us. It might simply be to restore our bodies to the size that He originally intended, or it may be something greater.

Yet only if we read His Word, believe His Word, apply His Word, and trust His Word, will God be able to harvest His seeds of righteousness in us.

Dear Lord, I trust in Your Word. May it find a fertile field in my heart, that Your seeds would be planted deep in me, and not return to You void. Amen.

WEEK TEN
DAY TWO

"For as the soil makes the sprout come up and garden causes seeds to grow, so the Sovereign Lord will make righteousness and praise spring up before all nations."

--Isa. 61:11

Jesus made references to trees, plants, fields, gardens, etc. when He spoke to the people – for many were common farmers, and could relate to parables and teachings about the land.

The land was where they lived – they could touch it, feel it, smell it, plant it, harvest it, and eat of its fruits.

Today, Jesus also speaks to us where we live – though our land may be concrete now, there is still soil in our hearts. We must open our hearts to Him as fertile soil into which He can plant the seed of His Word and His work.

Then... *"...as the soil makes the sprout come up,"* (in other words, as the roots grown deep in our spirit begin to sprout our good deeds for the Lord), *"...and a garden causes seeds to grow..."* (the garden being our lives planting seeds in others), then righteousness and praise *must* spring up!

Matthew 12:33 says, *"Make a tree good and its fruit will be good, or make a tree bad and its fruit will be bad, for a tree is recognized by its fruit."*

How can we be the good tree, from the good garden?

Jesus said in John 15:4, *"Remain in me and I will remain in you. No branch can bear fruit by itself; it must remain in the vine. Neither can you bear fruit unless you remain in me."*

Let Jesus, the Master Gardener, have His way with the soil of your heart, *"...so the Sovereign Lord will make righteousness and praise spring up before all nations."*

Dear Lord, let the soil of my heart be a harvest field for You. Let the fruit of my spirit bring forth Your righteousness. Amen.

WEEK TEN
DAY THREE

"Sow for yourselves righteousness, reap the fruit of unfailing love, and break up your unplowed ground; for it is time to seek the Lord, until he comes and showers righteousness on you."

--Hos. 10:12

Are there still areas of your heart that you have not submitted to the Lord? Unplowed ground which you have tried to keep hidden from others (and the Lord), hoping the rest of your brightly blooming garden will so occupy them that they won't see the unplowed ground?

Maybe you've even been successful in hiding this unplowed ground from others – but remind yourself that *nothing* is hidden from God's sight! He sees your unplowed ground, no matter how well-hidden from the rest of the world.

Maybe you are already sowing righteousness in your desert of testing with food – if so, that's great!

Maybe you are even reaping the fruit of unfailing love in your Christian walk – if so, that's wonderful!

BUT… God's Word says that you must also break up your *unplowed* ground. You are being disobedient if you hold *any* area back from the Lord.

This book is about a program of deliverance from bondage. *All* bondage – not just food.

Maybe God has already delivered you from the bondage to food – it could be that He's even delivered you from another area of bondage already. But it could also be that He now wants to deliver you from your *"unplowed ground"* – to be submissive to your spouse, to be free from fear, to let go of the past, to be delivered from your deepest bondage...

You must submit even this area of your garden to your Heavenly Father, the Master Gardener; *"for it is time to seek the Lord, until he comes and showers righteousness on you."*

Dear Lord, show me any "unplowed ground" I may still have, and help me to submit it to You, no matter how difficult it seems. Have Your way and deliver me from this deepest, hidden bondage. Amen.

WEEK TEN
DAY FOUR

"As the Father has loved me, so have I loved you. Now remain in my love. If you obey my commands, you will remain in my love, just as I have obeyed my Father's commands and remain in his love. I have told you this so that my joy may be in you and that your joy may be complete."

--Jn. 15:9-11

What a joy there is when we let go! What a complete joy there is in deliverance!

Jesus promises this joy to us when we let Him have His way in us – when we submit *every* area of our lives to Him, holding nothing back.

Remember the old bumper sticker, "Let Go and Let God?" What a simple concept, yet how strongly we resist it!

There's a joke that talks about a man over the edge of a cliff clinging tightly to a vine. He screamed for help, saying, "Is there anybody up there?"

A voice answered him, saying, "This is God. Have faith and let go."

The man hesitated, considering his situation, before he asked, "Is there anybody *else* up there?"

How tightly are you clinging to *your* vine? How afraid are you to let go that even when you hear the voice of God, you also ask, "Is there anybody *else* up there?"'

Jesus loves you. He wants His joy to be complete in you, and for your joy to be complete.

Yet He cannot give you this wonderful joy if you don't believe that He loves you, if you don't trust His love to protect you from falling.

He said that *if* you obey His commands, even as He obeyed God's commands, *then* you will remain in His love (remember those "If...Then's?"). And because *"love covers over a multitude of sins"* (1Peter 4:8)... by letting go and letting God have His way in you, your joy truly will be complete.

Dear Lord, I confess my reluctance to let go and let You have Your way in me. Give me the faith to let go of even those deepest areas of bondage, so that I might experience the joy of deliverance. Amen.

WEEK TEN
DAY FIVE

"Dear friends, do not be surprised at the painful trial you are suffering, as though something strange were happening to you. But rejoice that you participate in the sufferings of Christ, so that you may be overjoyed when his glory is revealed."

--1Pet. 4:12-13

Some of life's hardest lessons come with its deepest pain.

Having to face your deepest bondage may be the hardest thing you've ever done.

Yet your Heavenly Father, out of His great love for you, would have you even to experience this deepest pain now, so that later you would be overjoyed when His glory is revealed (and notice that it says *when*, and not *if!*).

If given the choice, none of us would willingly participate in suffering. Yet God's Word says to *rejoice* that we participate in the sufferings of Christ. Not just *willingly*, then, but *gladly* also.

Some of us even easily renounce Peter's denial, arrogantly claiming, "*I* could never deny Christ!" But could you bear His cross? Yet He doesn't even ask you to do that – He only asks you to bear your *own* cross!

Jesus said in Luke 9:23, *"If any man will come after me, let him deny himself and take up his cross daily, and follow me."* Can you do that?

Will you deny yourself this cross which you grasp so tightly on the ground, this painful trial you are suffering, to let *Jesus* help you carry it? Nay, even *deliver* you from it?

He's not even asking you to be obedient in this deliverance – He's only asking you to be *willing* to be obedient. Then His glory will truly be revealed in you.

Dear Lord, I repent of my fear of letting go. Help me to take up this cross so that nothing would prevent me from following after You. Amen.

WEEK TEN
DAY SIX

"So then, those who suffer according to God's will should commit themselves to their faithful Creator and continue to do good."

--1Pet. 4:19

How much do you trust God? Do you trust Him with this suffering?

You must make a choice – either you give it to God, or you keep it for yourself.

If you keep it for yourself, *you* are in control. Wouldn't you rather submit this suffering to God, and let *Him* be in control?

How many of you, as children, heard your parents say, "I never said it would be easy!"

Well, your Heavenly Father never said that committing yourself to Him would be easy, either. He did say that it would be worth it, though, according to Luke 9:24, when He said, *"For whoever wants to save his life will lose it, but whoever loses his life for me will save it."*

Maybe deliverance for you will not come with all the fireworks and revelation that it might for someone else.

For you, this deliverance could be a gradual thing – a matter of "continuing to do good," while, having committed yourself to God, He "works out" the rest, as He says in Romans 8:28:

"And we know that in all things God works for the good of those who love him, who have been called according to his purpose."

God only asks you to commit yourself to Him and continue to do good. Then the victory belongs to Him, for as it says in Proverbs 21:31, *"The horse is made ready for the day of battle, but victory rests with the Lord."*

Dear Lord, I commit myself to You. Help me to continue to do good, even as I trust in You and the victory You will bring out of this. Amen.

WEEK TEN
DAY SEVEN

"What then shall we say? That the Gentiles, who did not pursue righteousness, have obtained it, a righteousness that is by faith; but Israel, who pursued a law of righteousness, has not attained it. Why not? Because they pursued it not by faith but as if it were by works. They stumbled over the 'stumbling stone.'"

--Rom. 9:30-32

How could God's Word, in one breath, command us to *"continue to do good"* (1Peter 4:19), yet in another breath tell us that our works are wrong?

The key here is *faith*. The difference is the *"righteousness that is by faith."*

For although *"faith without works is dead"* (James 2:17), it is *obedience* that leads to righteousness, according to Romans 6:16, and that righteousness by *faith*.

According to Romans 3:22-24, *"This righteousness from God comes through faith in Jesus Christ to all who believe. There is no difference, for all have sinned and fall short of the glory of God, and are justified freely by his grace through the redemption that came by Christ Jesus."* By *His grace*, then, and *not* by *our works!*

"It does not, therefore, depend on man's desire or effort," says Romans 9:16, *"but on God's mercy."*

161

Many of us failed in worldly pursuits of weight loss, because we were trying to do it by our own works, our own effort, our own way.

In much the same way, many of us have failed in our spiritual walks because we have put that same emphasis on our own works, effort, and way... so that we, too, fell over the *"stumbling stone,"* because we *"pursued it not by faith but as if it were by works."*

Although God does command us to do good works, we must understand that our works will not justify our righteousness.

Only God's mercy can do that.

Dear Lord, I confess that I have lived by works and not by faith. Help me now to receive Your grace and mercy, so that I will no longer fall over the "stumbling stone." Amen.

WEEK ELEVEN
DAY ONE

"Yet he did not waver through unbelief regarding the promise of God, but was strengthened in his faith and gave glory to God, being fully persuaded that God had power to do what he had promised. This is why 'it was credited to him as righteousness.'"

--Rom. 4:20-22

Why was Abraham credited with righteousness?

Because he was a holy man, perfect in his obedience to God? Because his works bought his righteousness?

No! Abraham was credited by God with righteousness because *he believed God!*

That's it, no fancy "thee's" and "thou's" and "therefore's"... Just simply, as the saying goes, "God said it, I believe it, and that settles it."

Romans 4:20 tells us that Abraham *"did not waver in unbelief regarding the promise of God."*

Does that mean that he never struggled with unbelief, as we do, or only that *in* that unbelief he still didn't waver?

Abraham was *"fully persuaded that God had power to do what he had promised."*

Are you?

Has God given you a promise that you will be delivered from the bondage to food? Do you believe Him?

If God has, indeed, given you a promise – whether deliverance from food, or any other promise – you can expect that your faith will be tested regarding that promise. You might even be expected to be tried through unbelief.

But if, like Abraham, you do not waver through unbelief, you will be like him, who *"was strengthened in his faith and gave glory to God."*

Dear Lord, help me not to waver in my unbelief. I believe Your promise. Help me to be strengthened in my faith so that I can give glory to You. Amen.

WEEK ELEVEN
DAY TWO

"For if, by the trespass of the one man, death reigned through that one man, how much more will those who receive God's abundant provision of grace and of the gift of righteousness reign in life through the one man, Jesus Christ."

--Rom. 5:17

So if our own works cannot attain righteousness for us, and if this righteousness can only come by faith, how then can we hope to receive this righteousness at all?

Well, we can't – in and of ourselves, we can't! Just like we can't *save* ourselves.

However, we can receive the *gift* of salvation, just as we can receive the *gift* of righteousness, *"through the one man, Jesus Christ."*

Admitting that we can't do things our own way any more, or that our way won't work, frees us also to receive *"God's abundant provision of grace."* And what a freedom that is!

When death reigned in us through sin, didn't we also feel the heaviness of that weight on us?

Yet when we received deliverance through Christ, we are as "lighter" spiritually as our bodies are "lighter" (losing weight) in the physical.

Through God's grace, our burdens are lifted –
through His *abundant* grace we receive the gift of
righteousness!

What a freedom to know that we don't have to
obey a set of man-made rules, to diet, conforming
ourselves to the image of the advertising world, ever
again!

God Himself will deliver us from that, and that
freely, as we receive His gift of grace.

What a freedom to know that spiritually we
don't have to struggle with a set of man-made rules,
either, or a "spiritual diet," conforming ourselves to the
image of other Christians, instead of to Christ Himself.
We can freely receive the gift of righteousness.

*Dear Lord, I thank You for Your abundant grace and
the gift of righteousness. I praise You for deliverance
from man-made rules. Amen.*

WEEK ELEVEN
DAY THREE

"After beginning with the Spirit, are you now trying to attain your goal by human effort?"

--Gal. 3:3

Okay, back to basics: Led by the Spirit, you stepped out in faith.

The beginning was wonderful – buoyant, even! Then there was the sweet taste of success; the sheer joy of God's presence and grace in granting freedom from bondage.

Praise the Lord, you started losing weight! And it was *God's* way, not man's way.

Spirit-led, you continued through your desert of testing and remained firm in your resolve to continue walking God's way and not your own.

Then you reached that plateau (we all do). That time of testing where there may be no outward evidence of inward change, that time when you must go through a real testing of your obedience.

Will you still be faithful without being able to *see* the fruits of your faith? Proverbs 24:10 says, *"If you falter in times of trouble, how small is your strength."*

We all reach the crossroads, where we need to make a choice whether to remain obedient or to go back to our old ways. For some, you may even be like the Galatians, whom Paul chastised by saying, *"After beginning with the Spirit, are you now trying to attain your goal by human effort?"*

You may even be tempted to "hurry the process" by going back to one of your old diets (or trying a new one).

It is not by your own strength (Proverbs 24:10), nor your own effort (Galatians 3:3), that you will find success in your desert of testing. God says in Zechariah 4:6, *"'Not by might, nor by power, but by my Spirit,' says the Lord Almighty."*

After beginning with the Spirit, are *you* now trying to reach your goal your own way (by human effort)? If you are, then you must again make the decision to be obedient and let *God* deliver you through your desert of testing.

Dear Lord, I'm sorry I tried to do it my own way again. I know it's not by my might nor by my power, but only by Your Spirit that I will find victory. Amen.

WEEK ELEVEN
DAY FOUR

"Have you suffered so much for nothing – if it really was for nothing? Does God give you his Spirit and work miracles among you because you observe the law or because you believe what you heard?"

--Gal. 3:4-5

Have you reached a "dry place" in your desert? That "hard rock" place where it seems you'll never get past?

Are you beginning to wonder if you will *ever* reach your weight loss goal? Are you wondering if you have *"suffered so much for nothing – if it really was for nothing?"*

Could it be that in this "dry place," you are struggling again with the idea of obedience? Again having to make the choice between God's way and man's way (one of your old "quick-fix" diets)?

Then I ask you as Paul asked the Galatians, *"Does God give you his spirit and work miracles among you because you observe the law or because you believe what you heard?"*

Remember, you came to this place in the beginning by the Spirit's leading, and because the "man-made law" did *not* work for you! Why be tempted to go back to it now?

Remember how you felt when you first began this book – the hope you had – the faith on which you began your journey through the desert. No, you didn't come because you *"observe the law,"* but *"because you believe what you heard"* when the Spirit spoke to you.

Whether salvation was an instantaneous decision for you, or whether you struggled with it over time, you were still delivered unto salvation, weren't you?

You may even have already heard testimonies of others who had already found success through obedience to God – those who were finding freedom from bondage, *God's* way. And you believed what you heard.

This is not the time to fall back and return to old ways. This is the time to remember why you came, why you are here, and to persevere through this dry, hard time, holding to God's promise, *"because you believe what you heard."*

Dear Lord, help me to be strong and to continue in obedience to You, even as I am tempted to return to old ways. Amen.

WEEK ELEVEN
DAY FIVE

"It is for freedom that Christ has set us free. Stand firm, then, and do not let yourselves be burdened again by a yoke of slavery."

--Gal. 5:1

Usually about halfway through any journey, the weariness will set in.

Like children in the back seat of a car on a long-distance family trip, we ask, "Are we there yet?"

And, just like our earthly father, our Heavenly Father answers, "I'll let you know when we're there – just be patient."

Yes, it gets difficult for all of us, no matter which desert of testing, no matter what journey, no matter the goal – we all reach that halfway-plus point where the newness has worn off, the excitement has worn thin, and we are left with only the day-to-day seemingly mundane walk of obedience; that place of simply "standing firm."

Could it be that our excitement has waxed cold because we have lost sight of our goal?

Long-distance runners do not always see the finish line in front of them – it is only when they round that last bend that they actually have their goal in sight.

Yet for most of their journey, they keep the *vision* of that finish line in their mind, and thus they never truly do lose sight of their goal.

What *is* our goal, then? That "finish line" of which we must never lose sight? It is our *freedom!* For *"It is for freedom that Christ has set us free."*

God knew we would reach this point in our journey, so He gives us this encouragement in Galatians, to *stand firm.* He knew we would be tempted to go back to our old ways, or the "easy way," so He says to: *"Stand firm, then, and do not let yourselves be burdened again by a yoke of slavery."* He gently reminds us of the slavery waiting for us back in our own "Egypt," hoping we will continue on with Him to our own Promised Land ahead.

Dear Lord, it's so hard to keep that goal in mind when I'm tempted to take the easy way out. Strengthen my resolve to be obedient to Your way – help me to stand firm. Amen.

WEEK ELEVEN
DAY SIX

"But by faith we eagerly await through the Spirit the righteousness for which we hope."

--Gal. 5:5

Okay, let's recap. You've stepped out, *"beginning with the Spirit"* (Galatians 3:3)... You *"believe what you heard"* (Galatians 3:5)... You're standing firm, believing that *"it is for freedom that Christ has set us free"* (Galatians 5:1), so you have your finish line set in your "mind's-eye"...

But yet you ask yourself, "How do I get from here to there?"

Again our Heavenly Father has the answer for you – *by faith.* By faith *through the Spirit.* *"But by faith we eagerly await through the Spirit the righteousness for which we hope."* (Galatians 5:5)

It doesn't just say we wait, it says we wait *eagerly!* Again, the image of the children in the back seat of a long-distance car ride comes to mind – *eagerly awaiting;* anticipating that arrival at Grandma's, or Disneyland, or the beach – that is their hope.

What is *our* hope then? Where are we eagerly anticipating our journey to end? What is our "Disneyland?"

It is *righteousness*! *"We eagerly await through the Spirit the righteousness for which we hope."*

Just as Dad doesn't explain to the kids each step of the journey, but simply admonishes them to wait (*eagerly await*), so our Heavenly Father does not explain each step of this journey to us, but simply admonishes *us* to wait (*eagerly await*).

Dear Lord, I know I get as impatient as a child sometimes and ask, "Are we there yet?" Help me to be content with standing firm and eagerly awaiting instead of hurrying the journey. Amen.

WEEK ELEVEN
DAY SEVEN

"What good is it, my brothers, if a man claims to have faith but has no deeds? Can such faith save him?"

--James 2:14

The real test of faith is to love another in spite of their shortcomings – to choose to look beyond that person's physical imperfections and deep into their *character*, which is being spiritually perfected day by day.

This is the way the Lord loves us, the way He calls us to love others, and the way He calls us to love ourselves.

Our "deeds" consist of our "choices."

Each day you choose to be obedient to God's principles at work in your life, or you do not. Joshua 24:15 says, *"Choose for yourselves this day whom you will serve..."* not as if the walking out of our faith is an easy thing to accomplish, nor that it even comes naturally, but only that it exists in our choices – an act of the *will*.

Being a Christian means living in a paradoxical world, totally contrary to the "world" and its standards.

There used to be a saying, "If it feels good, do it!" But this is contrary to God's way, which asks us to be aware of our choices, and that the fruit of our choices should be "Godly fruit."

God does not ask us to be "religious" – in fact, the Pharisees were condemned for their outward religious acts of piety without the deep abiding faith within.

So it is not a matter of your acts bringing forth faith (or righteousness), but that your *faith* would bring forth good works.

James 2:18 ends with the words, *"Show me your faith without deeds, and I will show you my faith by what I do."*

Deep, abiding, godly faith cannot help but express itself in love.

Dear Lord, help me to love You, others, and myself, in a righteous manner. Help me each day to make the right choices, and to walk, by faith, in obedience to You. Amen.

WEEK TWELVE
DAY ONE

"In all my prayers for all of you, I always pray with joy because of your partnership in the gospel from the first day until now, being confident of this, that he who began a good work in you will carry it on to completion until the day of Christ Jesus."

--Phil. 1:6

Where is your confidence?

Many of us who have struggled with being overweight, or the bondage to food, have also battled with what the world calls "self-confidence" (or, rather, the lack of it).

Webster's dictionary calls confidence, "that in which faith is put; belief; trust."

The Lord never meant for us to battle with a lack of confidence, but it is a matter of where we direct our focus.

If "that in which faith is put" is Jesus Christ, we can, as Paul says, be *confident* that God will finish what He started in us.

If, however, "that in which faith is put" is our diet, our exercise program, or our own abilities, we will fail miserably in the area of confidence, because none of those things (including ourselves) has the ability to deliver us from bondage.

Only He who came *"to set the captives free"* (Isaiah 42:7) can deliver us from any bondage in which we find ourselves.

If your weight-loss walk has been faltering… if you have (again) been struggling with the issue of confidence or even (again) had the thought, "I just can't do it – I have no self-confidence…" then take heart!

God never meant you to be *self*-confident; He only meant you to be *Christ*-confident!

And, being Christ-confident, you can have "faith; belief; trust" in *His* desire and ability to complete the work *He* started in you.

Dear Lord, help me to be Christ-confident instead of self-confident, believing and trusting that You will complete that work which You've started in me. Amen.

WEEK TWELVE
DAY TWO

"Therefore, my dear friends, as you have always obeyed – not only in my presence, but now much more in my absence – continue to work out your salvation with fear and trembling, for it is God who works in you to will and to act according to his good purpose."

--Phil. 2:12-13

If you have questioned why this new way of thinking about things doesn't seem to be working for you any more, whether in the area of food, or any other bondage, check yourself – have you been acting the same way behind closed doors as you are when someone else is looking?

Paul commended the Philippians for their obedience, not just in his presence, but in his *absence*; and not just in his absence, but *"much more"* in his absence!

Some of us may even follow the new principles set out in this book when no one is looking, but do we do it to the *"much more"* extent for which Paul commended the Philippians?

Many of the "world's" 12-Step Programs have been successful because of the element of *accountability* to another person.

Many of us were in a weight-loss program that consisted of weekly meetings and were successful participants on meetings days/nights, when we were with the "fellowship of believers," yet we faltered in our obedience when left to ourselves.

Could it be because our emphasis has been on our *own* abilities, instead of working out our salvation *"in fear and trembling,"* focusing on *God's* ability to work *in* us *"to will and to act according to his good purpose?"*

Notice that the Scripture says according to *His* good purpose, and not what *we* decide His good purpose should be.

It is only by staying "Christ-confident" – not leaning only on ourselves or other friends also losing weight – that we can remain obedient whether anyone is looking or not.

Dear Lord, help me to stay Christ-confident instead of self-confident, and to remain obedient even when I am behind closed doors. Amen.

WEEK TWELVE
DAY THREE

"For everything that was written in the past was written to teach us, so that through endurance and the encouragement of the Scriptures we might have hope."

--Rom. 15:1

Have you ever come back from a vacation exhausted, exclaiming, "I need a vacation from my vacation!"? We try to cram so much into our short time-span of a vacation that it, many times, is even more "work" than the job we sought to escape!

How many of you are feeling that way about your new weight-loss walk? Have you put so much effort into *this* journey, that it has seemed like more "work" than the "job" from which you have been delivered?

Has this seemed more "labor" to you than "freedom?" And now, as the program winds down, are you exhausted, exclaiming, "I need a break from my weight-loss journey!"

STOP! This is a trick from the enemy to pull you back into old thinking. This way of weight loss is not something you "finish" and then "go back to work." It is a lifelong practice of Biblical principles; not just in the area of food, but in *all* areas of obedience to God.

If you are exhausted, if your desert has seemed too much like "work," and now you are looking forward to your "vacation," consider that your exhaustion may have come from some area(s) over which you have still not given God complete control.

If, at any time, we slip back into thinking that we can "do this on our own"… a kind of, "Thanks, God, for the teachings, but I can take it from here," we must tred carefully, for the chance is there to again become self-confident instead of Christ-confident.

Romans 15:1 tells us that *everything* that was written in the past was written to teach us. Do not forsake the journey – remember what you have learned. Why? Because God has called you to a walk not just of *obedience,* but of *endurance: "…so that through endurance and the encouragement of the Scriptures we might have hope."*

Dear Lord, I am so exhausted from this journey. Help me to find rest in You and in Your Word. Give me the encouragement I need to continue not just in obedience, but also in endurance. Amen.

WEEK TWELVE
DAY FOUR

"But blessed is the man who trusts in the Lord, whose confidence is in him."

--Jer. 17:7

Isn't it wonderful that we don't have to be concerned over our *own* self-confidence, but that we can rest from our journey in the arms of a loving Father, fully trusting in Him, having confidence in the One who loved us so much that He laid down His life for us?

What a wonderful God we serve! How far we've come from trusting in the *world* for our confidence, to trusting in the *Word* for our confidence! We can trust in Him who is the *author* of confidence!

Yes, the journey has been long (and not even completed yet), but our God is faithful to give us water for our thirst in the desert.

Some of you have found your Promised Land as far as deliverance from bondage to food – Praise the Lord! Yet now you feel God tugging at another chain of bondage (fear? submission? your calling? another addiction?) – and you find yourself crying out, "Wait, God! I just got this food-thing under control – I'm not ready to face the next desert yet!"

If this has been your thinking, then I would challenge you –do you really have this "food-thing" under control? If you do, then I would ask you, is it *your* control, or *God's* control? If you truly are in the Promised Land, then you are blessed in the hands of the Deliverer. You will be filled with the joy of freedom, and refreshed by the "living water" that brought you through your desert journey.

God may now be leading you toward deliverance from other bondages. If so, continue to walk in obedience to your Heavenly father, who wants only the best for you – to Him who would have you to be delivered from *everything* that stands in the way of an intimate relationship with Him.

Like Jeremiah, do not fear the coming trials, but claim instead that, *"Blessed is the man who trusts in the Lord, whose confidence is in Him."*

Dear Lord, I pray that You would stay in control of my life, instead of me. Thank You for bringing me this far, and help me to continue this journey with faith and trust only in You for my deliverance. Amen.

WEEK TWELVE
DAY FIVE

"I press on toward the goal to win the prize for which God has called me heavenward in Christ Jesus."

--Phil. 3:14

The hardest part of any race is when the "finish line" is in sight. By then, the runner is exhausted, thinking there is no more energy left to give. Yet, determined to win, he "presses on" toward the goal to get that prize. Adrenaline gives him a "second wind" (or third) – an extra measure of strength and energy to finish his race.

It is not unusual for us to be likened unto a runner. At this point, many of us *are* exhausted – the desert is not an easy place in which to travel. Many of us think we have no more energy left to give.

So how can we "press on" toward *our* "finish line?" By an extra measure of *God's grace.* God's grace is our adrenaline! His Holy Spirit is our "second wind" (or third), refreshing our spirits, as we continue on toward that goal.

Exhaustion comes from trying to do it all ourselves. God knew our desert of testing would be difficult, but it was never meant to bring us to the point of exhaustion… *unless* it is the exhaustion of our own resources.

There is an expression that says, "When you get to the end of *self,* you have found the beginning of

God." It is only when you truly have exhausted all your own natural resources, that you can fully rely on God's *unlimited* resources to help you finish your race and receive your prize.

As Paul told the Philippians, however, it was never *their* prize (nor is it *yours*) to begin with! *"I press on toward the goal to win the prize for which God has called me heavenward in Christ Jesus,"* he said. That prize for which *God* has called me! And not a prize of this world – a *heavenly* prize! And not for ourselves, but *in Christ Jesus!*

Praise the Lord, that He gives us abundantly *above* anything this world could offer us – our "prize" is eternal life! Whether, at this point, you've lost all the weight you wanted to lose or not, your Promised Land still awaits you in Heaven – your prize is to be with the One who traveled with you in the desert and who never left your side!

Dear Lord, thank You for staying with me through this journey. Whether my finish line is today or tomorrow, or not for a long time, help me to always keep in mind that the real prize comes in serving You, and serving You only. Amen.

WEEK TWELVE
DAY SIX

"Not that I have already obtained all this, or have already been made perfect, but I press on to take hold of that for which Christ Jesus took hold of me."

--Phil. 3:12

I remember thinking, at one point, that I had "failed." I hadn't lost the weight I wanted to lose fast enough, by my own standards. I had slipped back into the world's definition of success, thinking that since I hadn't lost all the weight as quickly as the magazines tell you that you can, that somehow I was a "failure." Oh, how my Heavenly Father gently rebuked me then.

I had made the mistake of judging my inward changes by my outward appearance – I had taken my eyes off Jesus, and the work He was doing in me, and was thinking I had failed because He somehow wasn't finished with me yet.

You've heard the expression, "Be patient – God's not finished with me yet!" Well, I had somehow equated "finished" with "being perfect."

What a treasure I received when God showed me Paul's words, *"Not that I have already obtained all this, or have been made perfect..."* "You mean, it's okay to not be perfect?" I thought. Whoops – there went the last of my high self-expectations!

It was hard for me to realize that this new way of weight loss God's way was not something you "finish," but is a lifestyle change instead, lasting forever. Especially since I had been a "successful dieter" in the past, finishing many programs – unfortunately, like many of you, I always gained the weight back and more, after "graduation" from the diet or program.

The walk of obedience is a *lifetime* walk. We will not "finish" until we die – our "graduation" will be in Heaven. But praise God for the journey *through* which we are learning obedience – *though* which we learn to fellowship with our Lord – *through* which we have learned to trust Him to meet all our needs, *through* which we have begun to be delivered from *all* our bondages! But, especially, that in our desert of testing, *though* which we come, we have a loving God who, never once, leaves us alone in our desert.

Dear Lord, I praise You for Your faithfulness. Even when I haven't felt You near me in this desert, I know You have still been there, helping me through. Continue with me now, as I make this desert walk a lifetime walk of obedience to You. Amen.

WEEK TWELVE
DAY SEVEN

"If you love me, you will obey what I command."
--Jn. 14:15
"I will not leave you as orphans; I will come to you."
--Jn. 14:18
"Whoever has my commands and obeys them, he is the one who loves me. He who loves me will be loved by my Father, and I too will love him and show myself to him."
--Jn. 14:21

If you love me… If you *love* me… If you love *me*… Jesus says. Do you love Him? Then do what He told you to do. Has He called you to continue this obedience journey? Then do so – and consider in your reluctance, that you may be called to be there for someone else, and not just yourself. If so, allow Him to use you.

Has God called you to a ministry? Then obey what He commands – whether that ministry is in the world, the church, or your own home, serving the needs of your family. Obey Him. Has He called you to teach what you have learned during this journey to others? Then obey Him. If you love Him, you will obey Him.

The principles taught in this book are *God's* principles – a lifetime walk of obedience to our Lord, who calls us into this walk to be His hands, His feet, His voice, to a dying world. Whether it is salvation to the unsaved, or deliverance from bondage for the believer, as Christ poured Himself out for us, so we must now pour ourselves out for others.

"If you love me, you will obey what I command," He says. And what is His command? *"Jesus replied, 'Love the Lord your God with all your heart and with all your soul and with all your mind.' This is the first and greatest commandment. And the second is like it: 'Love your neighbor as yourself.' All the Law and the Prophets hang on these two commandments.'" (Matt. 22:37-40)*

Do you love Him with all your heart (an undivided heart)? Do you love Him with all your soul (totally abandoned to the work of the Holy Spirit in you)? Do you love Him with all your mind (are you Christ-confident instead of self-confident)? Do you love yourself (can you accept yourself as "unfinished," yet not a "failure")? And can you love your neighbor as yourself (as Christ loved you and gave Himself up for you)?

Then GO. Continue your walk with God, obediently doing what He commands, knowing that He will not leave you as an orphan, but will come to you, and show Himself to you.

Dear Lord, I do want to love You with all my heart, soul, and mind. I want to serve You as You have called me to do, but I know I can't do this on my own. Help me, Lord, to love you deeper, live for You stronger, and serve You greater, than I ever have before. Amen.

"If you love me, you will obey what I command. And I will ask the Father, and he will give you another Counselor to be with you forever – the Spirit of truth. The world cannot accept him, because it neither sees him nor knows him. But you know him, for he lives with you and will be in you.

I will not leave you as orphans; I will come to you. Before long, the world will not see me anymore, but you will see me. Because I live, you also will live. On that day you will realize that I am in my Father, and you are in me, and I am in you.

Whoever has my commands and obeys them, he is the one who loves me. He who loves me will be loved by my Father, and I too will love him and show myself to him.

Then Judas (not Judas Iscariot) said, 'But Lord, why do you intend to show yourself to us and not to the world?'

Jesus replied, 'If anyone loves me, he will obey my teaching. My Father will love him, and we will come to him and make our home with him. He who does not love me will not obey my teaching. These words you hear are not my own; they belong to the Father who sent me.

All this I have spoken while still with you. But the Counselor, the Holy Spirit, whom the Father will send in my name, will teach you all things and will remind you of everything I have said to you.

Peace I leave with you; my peace I give you. I do not give to you as the world gives. Do not let your hearts be troubled and do not be afraid."

--Jn. 14:15-27